Iryna Lobanova

Acute disseminated encephalomyelitis

Iryna Lobanova

Acute disseminated encephalomyelitis

LAP LAMBERT Academic Publishing

Impressum / Imprint

Bibliografische Information der Deutschen Nationalbibliothek: Die Deutsche Nationalbibliothek verzeichnet diese Publikation in der Deutschen Nationalbibliografie; detaillierte bibliografische Daten sind im Internet über http://dnb.d-nb.de abrufbar.

Alle in diesem Buch genannten Marken und Produktnamen unterliegen warenzeichen-, marken- oder patentrechtlichem Schutz bzw. sind Warenzeichen oder eingetragene Warenzeichen der jeweiligen Inhaber. Die Wiedergabe von Marken, Produktnamen, Gebrauchsnamen, Handelsnamen, Warenbezeichnungen u.s.w. in diesem Werk berechtigt auch ohne besondere Kennzeichnung nicht zu der Annahme, dass solche Namen im Sinne der Warenzeichen- und Markenschutzgesetzgebung als frei zu betrachten wären und daher von jedermann benutzt werden dürften.

Bibliographic information published by the Deutsche Nationalbibliothek: The Deutsche Nationalbibliothek lists this publication in the Deutsche Nationalbibliografie; detailed bibliographic data are available in the Internet at http://dnb.d-nb.de.

Any brand names and product names mentioned in this book are subject to trademark, brand or patent protection and are trademarks or registered trademarks of their respective holders. The use of brand names, product names, common names, trade names, product descriptions etc. even without a particular marking in this work is in no way to be construed to mean that such names may be regarded as unrestricted in respect of trademark and brand protection legislation and could thus be used by anyone.

Coverbild / Cover image: www.ingimage.com

Verlag / Publisher:
LAP LAMBERT Academic Publishing
ist ein Imprint der / is a trademark of
OmniScriptum GmbH & Co. KG
Heinrich-Böcking-Str. 6-8, 66121 Saarbrücken, Deutschland / Germany
Email: info@lap-publishing.com

Herstellung: siehe letzte Seite /
Printed at: see last page
ISBN: 978-3-659-75821-8

Clinic-neurological characteristics of acute disseminated encephalomyelitis, its treatment and prediction of transformation into multiple sclerosis.

TABLE OF CONTENTS

Introduction.

Increasing the efficacy of the treatment of patients with acute disseminated encephalomyelitis (ADEM) remains an actual problem for clinical neurology. ADEM is an autoimmune disease characterized by presence of inflammation and demyelination foci, having been caused by infectious disease or vaccination, in the central nervous system [1, 2, 3, 4, 5, 6]. The following infections may be the triggering factors for ADEM: viral factors (measles, rubella, mumps, parainfluenza viruses [7, 8, 9, 10, 11], hepatitis A and B [7, 12, 13], whooping cough, tetanus [7, 14, 15], Epstein-Barr virus, cytomegalovirus and bacterial factors (Mycoplasma pneumonie [7, 16, 17, 18, 19, 20], Campylobacter [7, 21, 22, 23], Borrelia Burgdogferi [7, 24, 25], Leptospira, Chlamydia, Legionella, B -hemolytic streptococcus group A [7, 26, 27, 28]. However, in most cases there is evidence of a nonspecific upper respiratory tract infection and there is no serologic evidence of pathogen [7, 24, 29, 30]. Vaccines that may lead to ADEM development include vaccines against influenza, measles, hepatitis B, rabies, tetanus, chicken pox [7, 26, 31, 32, 33, 34]. There are also cases of spontaneous development of the disease [7, 35, 36, 37].

Infectious factor is closely associated with the pathogenesis of ADEM, but it is not localized in the central nervous system or spinal fluid, virus replication in brain cells does not arise. It is not clear how it leads to the development of demyelinating disease that is why there is a hypothesis of molecular mimicry [7, 24]. According to this theory, some infectious agents have peptides similar to immune-dominant epitope of myelin basic protein (MBP). It means that these infectious pathogens can activate T-cells that are autoreactive to MBP in case if phenotype of certain antigens is present in HLA (Human Leukocyte Antigen). It is known that HLA-system has two classes of molecules: I (A, B, C) is expressed on all nuclear cells and II (DR, DQ, DP) is expressed on cells involved in antigen presentation. Currently, ADEM is associated with genotype DRB1*01 and DRB1*03(017). But it is not clear why so many infectious agents can cause one disease. A possible explanation for this is another hypothesis – direct penetration of neurotropic virus in the central nervous system (CNS) opens brain antigens, previously closed to the immune system, and myelin proteins, causing an inflammatory response that leads to immune-mediated demyelination [15, 24].

The development of experimental models, including experimental allergic encephalomyelitis (EAE), has made an important contribution to the understanding of immunopathogenesis of acute disseminated encephalomyelitis [7, 24]. EAE in Theiler's virus model is an autoimmune condition that can be reproduced in animals by administering myelin antigens such as MBP, proteolipid protein and glycoprotein of oligodendrocytes [15], causing primary systemic impulse in autoimmune reaction appearance. Penetrating into peripheral blood, antigen is phagocyted by macrophages that present it on their surface as a part of receptors of main complex of histocompatibility (HLA), after that the antigen is recognized by CD4 + T-cells-helpers. They, in their turn, stimulate the formation of proinflammatory cytokines, resulting in lesion of the blood-brain barrier (BBB), after that autoreactive T-cells with CD4-phenotype to the antigens - myelin basic protein (MBP), proteolipid protein or myelin-oligodendrocyte glycoprotein get into the central nervous system from peripheral blood. In brain tissue they are reactivated by cytotoxic T-cells, B-cells, macrophages and glial cells, and enhance cascade of immunopathological reactions: expression of adhesion molecules and antigen-presenting molecules (HLA-molecules) to the endothelium of the brain vessels and gliocytes; increased production of proinflammatory cytokines – gamma-interferon, tumor-necrosis factor-alpha (TNFα), interleukins (IL-1, SHL-2, IL-12, IL-15), autoantibodies of proteases, chemokines, free radicals, nitric oxide; decreased synthesis of proinflammatory cytokines - IL-4, IL-10, beta-interferon. It leads to violation of BBB permeability, activation of B cells and all components of humoral immunity, complement system and monocytes/macrophages [15]. These autoimmune and pathobiochemical reactions cause formation of disseminated perivascular foci of inflammation, especially around capillary, venous structures (small and medium), causing an inflammatory reaction cascade, destruction of myelin (demyelination), lesion of axons. Thus, the pathogenesis of acute disseminated encephalomyelitis has autoimmune nature and is accompanied by typical pathological changes.

The criteria necessary for the diagnosis of acute disseminated encephalomyelitis are given in the book of Harris C. et al, 2007 [4]. In 2007, the International Pediatric Multiple Sclerosis Study Group defined ADEM as "the first clinical event with a poly-symptomatic encephalopathy, with acute or subacute onset, showing focal or multifocal hyperintense lesions predominantly affecting the CNS white matter"[7, 4]. This definition shows how difficult it may be to differentiate ADEM from a multiple sclerosis at an early stage [38].Magnetic resonance imaging can help in differentiating ADEM from multiple sclerosis although many features look the same. In ADEM, lesions are typically extensive but poorly defined. They are mainly found in the white matter but can extend to the deep gray matter. Multiple sclerosis lesions are commonly found in the periventricular white matter and corpus callosum and are less likely to involve the gray matter [38].

According to the recent studies of International Pediatric Multiple Sclerosis Study Group (IPMS), ADEM is regarded as polysymptomatic disease with multifocal lesion of CNS. Encephalopathy and disorders of consciousness are part of the presentation [39]. Some authors consider ADEM as polysymptomatic demyelinating inflammatory disease which is characterized by acute or subacute onset, no data about preceding lesion of CNS, significant improvement of patient's condition after the treatment [39, 40]. Also ADEM is characterized by the signs of systemic inflammatory response (headache, dizziness, nausea, fever, myalgia), appearing a few days – weeks after the infectious disease (so-called latent period) [41, 42].

In most cases, ADEM is characterized by the monophasic course accompanied by considerable variations in the duration of the disease and period of convalescence of the patient. However, there are also possible relapses of ADEM that have already been known since 1932, as described by van Bogaert, who published the paper "ADEM with relapses" [36, 43]. ADEM relapses can be considered as a multiphasic course of this disease or its transformation into multiple sclerosis (MS) (according to the McDonald Criteria) [43, 44-50]. The relapse rate of ADEM has been described, ranging from 5.5% to 24% [43, 51-58].

New clinical symptoms appearing three months after initial signs of this disease are considered as a relapse of ADEM. In case of the disease relapse, the pathological process comprises new parts of brain and/or spinal cord (which is usually confirmed by clinical investigations and neurovisual methods) [43].

If the relapse appears in a short time interval after initial signs and is combined with further infection or cancelled hormonal therapy, the term multiphasic disseminated encephalomyelitis (MDEM) should be used [12, 43, 58]. In the opinion of researchers , MDEM is characterized by poly-symptomatic manifestations of this disease, availability of demyelination nidi in Magnetic resonance imaging (MRI) data, mainly in subcortical parts of brain, in less degree located periventricularly, with total or partial disappearance of foci during the convalescent period [43, 59]. The multiphasic course of disseminated encephalomyelitis can be diagnosed in the case of disease relapse appearance at least 3 months after its initial presentation [12, 36, 43, 57, 59]. Appearance of new clinic symptoms and new foci in MRI data 12 to 18 months after the primary episode of the disease is indicative of its possible transformation into multiple sclerosis (MS) (according to the McDonald Criteria) [43, 50, 60]. Relapses of acute disseminated encephalomyelitis are called multiphase course of the disease [24, 43]. Therefore treatment of acute disseminated encephalomyelitis must be aimed at reducing intensity of neurological impairment and prevention of the disease relapses.

There is a lack of controlled clinical trials and no proven standard treatment for ADEM. Most treatment options are based on empirical and observational evidence. Once ADEM is diagnosed and acute infectious etiology is excluded, treatment should be instituted as soon as possible [43, 61, 62].

There is a lack of evidence-based, prospective clinical trial data for the management of ADEM [63]. As far as development of the disease is caused by autoimmune response, patients are recommended pathogenetic immunosuppressive therapy aimed at suppression of the immune response to infectious agent or vaccination with the high doses of corticosteroids [43, 64-68]. Hormone therapy is also recommended due to its ability to block or modify the course of experimental allergic encephalomyelitis. In addition to its anti-inflammatory and immunosuppressive action, hormone therapy restores the function of blood-brain barrier, activates phagocytosis and immunoglobulin synthesis. Intravenous administration of corticosteroids over a period of several days followed by their peroral administration is considered to be the most common treatment scheme [43, 63, 69-74]. However, in cases where the efficacy of pulse-therapy with corticosteroids is insufficient, intravenous administration of immunoglobulin is used [43, 75-84]. Plasmapheresis method is also used for the treatment of patients with the diagnosis of ADEM [43, 63, 84-89]. However, the effectiveness of these treatments (glucocorticoids, intravenous immune globulin, and plasma exchange) for ADEM has not been definitively confirmed, as there are no prospective clinical trial data to determine optimal treatment, including dose or duration.

The **aim** of the study was:

1.   To assess the cognitive functions in patients with acute disseminated encephalomyelitis.

2.   To assess the degree of psychosocial and physical function impairment in patients diagnosed with acute disseminated encephalomyelitis and to identify the spheres of life affected by the disease the most.

3.   To determine the prognostic risk factors of development of the multiphase course in disseminated encephalomyelitis.

4.   To determine the prognostic risk factors of development of transformation of ADEM into multiple sclerosis

5.   To assess the prognostic significance of clinical and paraclinical indices for different types of acute disseminated encephalomyelitis course and its transformation into multiple sclerosis.

6.   To analyze the efficacy of intravenous immunoglobulin as therapeutic option in the treatment of patients with ADEM.

Methods:

We have examined 101 patients diagnosed with acute disseminated encephalomyelitis, 66 women and 35 men, aged 15- 53 (average age 32 ± 0.4). All the patients were being treated at the Kiev city centre of multiple sclerosis (Kiev city hospital number 4, Alexandrovskaya City Clinical Hospital, Kiev city, Ukraine). The diagnosis of ADEM was based on neurological examination, MRI of the brain and CSF analysis. All ADEM patients met the recently published diagnostic criteria [4]. The onset of disease in all patients was acute with evident disseminated lesion of central nervous system, increase of neurological deficit was observed during the short period of time (hours – days) and sudden development of encephalopathy. All patients underwent magnetic resonance imaging (MRI) studies of the brain and / or of the spinal cord to detect the location of the lesions of demyelination, lesion-load and size. The neurological status was assessed by Kurtzke an Expanded Disability Status Scale (EDSS) and Functional Systems Scores (FSS) [90]. Based on a standard neurological examination, the 7 functional systems (plus "other") are rated. These ratings are then used in conjunction with observations and information concerning gait and use of assistive devices to rate the EDSS. Each of the FSS is an ordinal clinical rating scale ranging from 0 to 5 or 6. The EDSS is an ordinal clinical rating scale ranging from 0 (normal neurologic examination) to 10 (death due to MS) in half-point increments. The FSS include pyramidal, cerebellar, brainstem, sensory, bowel and bladder, visual, cerebral (or mental), and other. The average point according to EDSS scale in patients with acute disseminated encephalomyelitis was 2.5±0.8 points. All patients were treated with hormonal pulse-therapy, using methylprednisolone in the dose of 500-1000 mg daily in 200 ml of isotonic sodium chloride solution (within 5 days).

All the patients were under observation for 3 years. If during this period (2 years) no relapse of demyelination disease was detected, it was interpreted it as the monophasic type of the ADEM course. In the case when disease relapses appeared, having the signs of disseminated encephalomyelitis from the clinical viewpoint and after neuro-visual patient examination, it was considered as the multiphasic option of the disease course. In the case of clinically confirmed multiple sclerosis (in accord with the McDonald criteria [50]), we interpreted it as transition of ADEM into multiple sclerosis.

According to the decision of the Ethics Committee of the O.O. Bogomolets National Medical University (Kyiv city, Ukraine), the investigations described in these articles have been carried out according to modern scientific standards. All patients signed informed consent form. There have been provided the measures ensuring safety of the patients, respect of their rights and dignity as well as moral and ethical standards in accordance with the human rights principles of the Declaration of Helsinki. Ethics Committee does not have any objections against publishing these articles (protocol number 48 dated 29.09.2010.)

The characteristics of cognitive functions in patients with acute disseminated encephalomyelitis.

The clinical picture of acute disseminated encephalomyelitis is characterized not only by a variety of neurological disorders, but also by disorders of higher cortical functions [7]. Disorders of higher cognitive functions often remain undetected during routine examination of patients and the use of specialized neuropsychological tests enables timely diagnosis of cognitive disorders. According to some authors, the vast majority of patients with ADEM have disorders of higher cortical functions of various severity [7, 91]. The sequelae of cognitive disorder include negative impact on daily life activities, employment, social functioning and relations. Neuropsychological examinations can be conducted for detecting cognitive changes, monitoring treatment effects, characterizing deficit of rehabilitation planning or documenting the range of patient's impairment for guiding decisions regarding disability.

The assessment of cognitive impairment was carried out in 67 patients with ADEM (28 male and 39 female, aged 16 – 50, mean age - 31.6 $\pm$2.3). At the beginning of the study cognitive functions were also assessed in 15 (8 male and 7 female) healthy, age matched control subjects (average age 32.5 $\pm$ 0.7years) with no systemic or neurological diseases. Patients of both clinical groups performed the same neuropsychological tests that enabled evaluation of short-term and long-term visual and auditory memory, various parameters of attention as well as ability to concentrate, orientation in time and space.

The "memory for numbers" and "memory for words" methods enabled evaluation of short-term and long-term visual memory. The patients were shown 20 numbers (or words) for over 30 seconds and then attempted to

8

recall them (immediately and after 1 hour). Method of 10 words memorizing included evaluation of short-term and long-term auditory memory. The patients were read 10 words, which were not related semantically, 7 times within 30 seconds. Each time the patients were asked to repeat the words immediately (assessment of short-term memory) and one hour later (assessment of long-term memory). California Verbal Learning Test [92] and Symbol Digit Modalities Test [93] were used to to measure key constructs in cognitive psychology such as repetition learning, serial position effects, semantic organization, intrusions, and proactive interference. MMSE (Mini - Mental State Examination) [94] enabled assessment of verbal learning and delayed recall, sustained attention and concentration as well as memory, attention and orientation in time and space.

In the statistical analysis the t-test was used for two-group comparisons of the cognitive functions of persons with acute disseminated encephalomyelitis and healthy individuals. Five percent for two tailed tests was chosen as the level of significance. Association between the severity of cognitive impairment according to the results of neuropsychological tests and EDSS scale score as well as the size of demyelination lesions on MRI were evaluated with Spearman rank correlation analysis.

Demographic and clinical data are shown in Table 1 and Table 2.

Table 1. Demographic and clinical profile of participants

Variables	Number of patients (%)
Overall numbers (%)	67 (100%)
Baseline age, (mean±SD) years	31.6 +2.3
Gender	
Men	28 (42)
Women	39 (58%)
Race	
White	67 (100%)
Educational attainment (years)	16.1±0.24
>=12 years	61 (91%)
<12 years	6 (9%)
Medical comorbidities	
Depression	-
Other psychiatric disorders	-
Hypertension	3
Diabetes mellitus	-
Hyperlipidemia	-

Atrial fibrillation	-
Cigarette smoking	5
Disability level according to the EDSS scale, points	2.5±0.8 points.

Table 2. Clinical presentation of patients with ADEM.

Variables	Number of patients (%)
Prior infection	4 (5,97%)
Prior immunization	4 (5,97%)
Polysymptomatic presentation	60 (89,6%)
Monosymptomatic presentation	7 (10,1 %)
Motor disturbances	57 (85,1 %)
Numbness/abnormal sensation	29 (43,3%)
Brain stem symptoms	11 (16,4%)
Unilateral optic neuritis	6 (8,95%)
Bilateral optic neuritis	1 (1,5%)
Cerebellar symptoms	48 (71,6%)
Encefalitis	5 (7,5%)
Myelitis	5 (7,5%)
Encephalopathy	63 (94,0%)
Seizures	17 (25,4%)

Taking into consideration the case history, significant negative impact of the disease on cognitive functions was subjectively noted by 23 (34%) patients of the main group. Patients with ADEM showed significantly worse results in performing the tests aimed to study cognitive functions compared to those of healthy individuals (control) (Table 3).

Table 3. Results of short-term and long-term memory study in patients with ADEM

Tests			Main group	Control group
"Memory for numbers" method	short-term	quantity of numbers	7.32±0.63*	13.6±0.49
		points	3.44±0.3*	6.45±0.22
	long-term	quantity of numbers	2.64±0.44*	9.3±0.54
		points	1.24±0.19*	4.4±0.28

"Memory for words" method	short-term	quantity of words	9.6±0.55*	13.04±0.28
		points	4.44±0.29*	8.2±0.7
	long-term	quantity of words	2.4±0.52*	8.4±0.25
		points	1.16±0.23*	3.45±0.11
"10 words memorizing" method		quantity of words	34.6±1.5*	42.7±1
		points	6.24±0.25^	7.4±0.2
California Verbal Learning Test		long term verbal recall	12. 3±1.9^	14.6±1.1
		Long term recognition	14.3±1.2	15.5±1.1
Symbol Digit Modalities Test			54.5±10.2	57.8±9.6
MMSE, points			27.02±0.24*	29.9±0.04

Note. * - Reliability of indices difference between groups of patients is P <0.001,

^ - reliability of indices difference between groups of patients is P <0.01.

Magnetic resonance tomography changes in all the patients constituted presence of demyelination foci – hyperintensive in T2-weighted image and hypointensive in T1-weighted image with the size 7 ± 0,6 mm. Size of single foci of demyelinization (28.8%) was 9.8 ± 1.75 mm, of multiple ones (84.8%) – 4.4 ± 0.4 mm.

Localization and frequency of brain lobes lesions in patients with ADEM accompanied by cognitive disorders is shown in Table 4 and 5.

Table 4. The frequency of demyelinating process lesion of different lobes of the brain in patients with ADEM

Lobe of the brain	Frequency of lesion, in %
Periventricular	72
Frontal lobes of hemispheres	33.6
Parietal lobes of hemispheres	28.8
Cerebellum	28.8
Subcortical	25.6
Pons	25.6
Thalamus	20
Semioval centres	19.2

Internal capsule	18
Temporal lobes of hemispheres	14.4
Corona radiate	14.4
Basal ganglia	12.8
Brainstem	6.4
Cerebral peduncle	6.4
Medulla oblongata	6.4
Occipital lobe	3.2

Table 5. The frequency of combined demyelinating process lesions of different lobes of the brain in patients with ADEM

Lobe of the brain	Frequency of lesion, in %
Periventricular and pons	20.8
Parietal and frontal lobes of hemispheres	19.2
Periventricular and parietal lobes of the brain	16
The frontal lobes of hemispheres and cerebellum	12.8
Subcortical and frontal lobes of hemispheres	11.2
Cerebellum and pons	11.2
Periventricular, frontal and parietal lobes of the brain	9.6
Periventricular, cerebellum and pons	8
Periventricular, frontal and temporal lobes of hemispheres	6.4
Periventricular, subcortical and cerebellum	6.4

We analyzed the correlation between the severity of cognitive impairment according to the results of neuropsychological tests and EDSS scale score (Table 6) as well as the size of demyelination lesions on MRI.

Table 6. Correlation analysis between the results of neuropsychological tests in patients with ADEM, age of patients and number of points according to EDSS scale.

Tests			Number of points according to EDSS scale	Degree of reliability
"Memory for numbers" method	short-term	Quantity of numbers	-0.2	P>0.05
		points	-0.13	P>0.05

	long-term	Quantity of numbers	-0.22	P>0.05
		points	-0.29	P>0.05
"Memory for words" method	short-term	Quantity of numbers	-0.13	P>0.05
		points	-0.34	P>0.05
	long-term	Quantity of numbers	-0.54	P<0.05
		points	-0.57	P<0.05
"10 words memorizing" method		Quantity of numbers	-0.52	P<0.05
		points	-0.48	P<0.05
California Verbal Learning Test		Long term verbal recall	-0.4	P<0.05
		Long term recognition	-0.4	P<0.05
Symbol Digit Modalities Test			0.02	P>0.05
MMSE			-0.32	P>0.05

There was statistically significant inverse relationship between short-term memory and attention, as assessed by the results of "10 words memorizing" (correlation coefficient r = -0.48; P <0.05), long-term auditory memory, as assessed by the results of "memory for words" (correlation coefficient r = -0.57; P <0.01), verbal learning and delayed recall, as assessed by the results of "California Verbal Learning Test", and the degree of disability according to EDSS scale score (correlation coefficient r = -0.4; P <0.05). Correlation analysis revealed no relation between the severity of cognitive impairment according to the results of neuropsychological tests and the size of demyelination foci on MRI. There was statistically significant inverse relationship between verbal learning and delayed recall, as assessed by the results of "California Verbal Learning Test" and lesion load of demyelinating process in frontal lobes of hemispheres (correlation coefficient r = - 0.5; p <0.05).

Analysis of the obtained results showed that patients with ADEM had significantly lower cognitive scores of cognitive functions such as short and long term visual and auditory memory, verbal learning and delayed recall, sustained attention and concentration as well as memory, attention and orientation in time and space. There was statistically significant inverse relationship between short-term memory and attention, long-term auditory memory, verbal learning and delayed recall and the degree of disability according to EDSS scale score.

It has been found that the severity of neuropsychological impairment correlated with the severity of neurological dysfunction in patients with ADEM. Demyelination foci in patients with cognitive disorders are most often localized to the periventricular regions in the frontal and parietal lobes, and in the cerebellum; where multiple demyelinating lesions are often observed.

The sequelae of cognitive disorders include negative impact on daily life activities, employment, social functioning and relations. Therapeutic correction of cognitive disorders in case of carrying out treatment-rehabilitation measures in patients with acute disseminated encephalomyelitis will improve the quality of life of patients.

A general assessment of the functional impact of acute disseminated encephalomyelitis.

Long-term disability in patients with acute disseminated encephalomyelitis is caused not only by neurological deficiency, but also by the difficulties with social and psychological adaptation [41]. Together with neurological condition, a very important role in clinical characteristics of the disease belongs to psychosocial disorders, as well as to patients' subjective perception of the disease symptoms that has the impact on their quality of life. Quality of life is impaired in ADEM in part due to physical disability. ADEM can diminish quality of life by interfering with the ability to work, pursue leisure activities, and carry on usual life roles. Symptoms that affect quality of life in patients with ADEM may include impaired mobility, fatigue, depression, pain, spasticity, cognitive impairment, sexual dysfunction, bowel and bladder dysfunction, vision and hearing problems, seizures. Polymorphic clinical features of ADEM significantly affect the quality of life of patients with this diagnosis – that was the main reason of carrying out this research.

We have examined 45 patients diagnosed with acute disseminated encephalomyelitis, 10 men and 35 women, aged 15- 53 (average age 32 ± 0.4). In order to assess the impact of the disease on the daily life of patients to the most full extent a survey was conducted with the use of tests: "Functional Limitation Profile" and "Sickness Impact Profile – 68" [95, 96]. All the patients were interrogated according to these tests after the acute period of disease – disappearance of encephalopathy phenomenon, i.e. disappearance of acute manifestations of the disease.

"Functional Limitation Profile" test helped to assess the change of patient's behavior in case of acute disseminated encephalomyelitis in 12 categories of life activity: "walk", "body care and motion", "movement", "household activity", "leisure and entertainments", "social interaction",

"emotions", "clarity of mind", "sleep and rest", "food", "communication",
"work". While carrying out "Sickness Impact Profile - 68" test, functional
condition of patients was assessed in 6 categories of life activity. "Somatic
autonomy" category reflected the extent of help that the patient requires
when performing everyday activities (dressing up, standing, walking, eating
etc). "Mobility control" category characterized the degree of control of
motion functions, including walking and actions with hands. "Psychic
autonomy and communication" category described behavior, connected with
mental functions and verbal communication. "Mobility degree" category
included the ways the disease limits household and professional activity.
"Social Behavior" category reflects social sphere of activity. "Emotional
stability" category reflects disease impact on the emotional sphere. All items
are scored dichotomously (no=0, yes =1). Points then were summed. A
higher point meant a worse quality of life.

There were no control subjects (without systemic or neurological
diseases), because according to the "Functional Limitation Profile" and
"Sickness Impact Profile – 68" tests no values are considered "normal", and
these tests are used only in subjects with certain diseases, not in healthy
individuals.

Statistical analysis of the results was made with the use of Stata 12.
Generalized characteristic of the investigated indices is represented by the
arithmetic mean (X). Variability of parameters was assessed by standard
deviation. The correlation between the degree of functional limitation in
patients with ADEM according to the results of the "Functional Limitation
Profile" and "Sickness Impact Profile – 68" tests and the size of
demyelination foci on MRI was evaluated with Pearson coefficient
correlation analysis. For comparative analysis there was used t-test (five
percent for two tailed tests was chosen as the level of significance) and $\chi 2$
test ($\alpha=0.05$, two sided).

Demographic and clinical data are shown in Table 7 and Table 8.

Table 7. Demographic and clinical profile of participants

Variables	Number of patients (%)
Overall numbers (%)	45 (100%)
Baseline age, (mean±SD) years	32 ± 0.4
Gender	
Men	10 (22%)
Women	35 (78%)
Race	

White	45 (100%)
Educational attainment (years)	16.1±0.24
>=12 years	42 (93%)
<12 years	3 (7%)
Medical comorbidities	
Depression	-
Other psychiatric disorders	-
Hypertension	3
Diabetes mellitus	-
Hyperlipidemia	-
Atrial fibrillation	-
Cigarette smoking	5
Immunosuppressing states	-
Immunodeficiency states	-
Immunosuppressive therapy prior to disease onset	-
Socioeconomic state	middle-income
Disability level according to the EDSS scale, points	2.5±0.8 points.

Table 8. Clinical presentation of patients with ADEM.

Variables	Number of patients (%)
Prior infection	2(4.4%)
Prior immunization	2(4.4%)
Polysymptomatic presentation	40(8.9%)
Monosymptomatic presentation	5(11.1%)
Motor disturbances	32(71.1%)
Numbness/abnormal sensation	18(40.0%)
Brain stem symptoms	8(17.8%)
Unilateral optic neuritis	4(8.9%0
Bilateral optic neuritis	1(2.2%)
Cerebellar symptoms	27(60.0%)
Encefalitis	3(6.7%)
Myelitis	2(4.4%)
Encephalopathy	43(95.6%)
Seizures	13(28.9%)

In all the patients, MRI detected foci of demyelination – hyperintensities on T2-weighted image and hypointensities on T1-weighted image (the size of $7 ± 0.6$ mm). Localization and frequency of lesions of the brain areas was the following: periventricular area – 72%, frontal lobes of hemispheres – 33.6%, parietal lobes – 28.8%, cerebellum – 28.8%, subcortical area – 25.6%, pons – 25.6%, thalamus – 20% , semioval centers –19.2%, internal capsule – 18%, temporal lobes – 14.4%, corona radiate – 14.4%, basal ganglia – 12.8%, brainstem – 6.4%, cerebral peduncle – 6.4%, medulla oblongata – 6.4%, occipital lobes – 3.2%.

Therefore, in patients with ADEM demyelination foci were located mostly periventricularly, less frequently they were detected in frontal and parietal lobes of the brain hemispheres and cerebellum. Brainstem, cerebral peduncle, medulla oblongata and occipital lobe were least commonly impaired. Perifocal edema around foci of demyelination was present in 27 patients (60% of cases). We found no statistically significant link between the degree of functional limitation in patients with ADEM according to the results of the "Functional Limitation Profile" and "Sickness Impact Profile - 68" tests and the size of demyelination foci on MRI (correlation coefficient $r = 0.01$; $P > 0.05$). However, we detected statistically significant relationship between the degree of functional limitation in patients with ADEM according to the results of the "Functional Limitation Profile" and "Sickness Impact Profile - 68" tests and the number of demyelination foci according to MRI data (correlation coefficient $r = 0.5$; $P < 0.05$) and the degree of disability on the EDSS (correlation coefficient $r = 0.7$; $P < 0.05$). Severity of neurologic deficit (assessed on the EDSS) and an increase in the number of demyelination foci on MRI have a negative impact on patients' self-assessment of their quality of life.

Assessment of the functional impact of acute disseminated encephalomyelitis according to the "Functional Limitation Profile" test data.

While conducting the "Functional Limitation Profile" test the functional condition changes were present in all the patients. The frequency of functional limitations is shown in Table 9 and Fig. 1. Patients with a diagnosis of acute disseminated encephalomyelitis showed the impairment of functional condition most often in 4 categories: "work", "leisure and entertainment", "social interaction" and "household activity".

Table 9. Assessment (in points) of the disease impact on the functional condition of patients according to the "Functional Limitation Profile" test data.

Behavior categories	Average point	Total point	Maximum possible point	% in relation to the maximum possible point
Walk	208±18	7700	45270	17
Body care and motion	282±42	11014	86715	13
Movement	186±14	4081	37715	11
Household activity	224±23	8965	30825	29

Leisure and entertainments	186±10	7813	17235	45
Social interaction	295±31	12093	58005	21
Emotions	142±7	2277	31185	7
Clarity of mind	273±20	9826	26595	37
Sleep and rest	129±6	2242	31770	7
Food	34	544	30825	2
Communication	94±4	1034	23400	4
Work	186±13	7987	26000	31

Assessment of the functional impact of acute disseminated encephalomyelitis according to the "Sickness Impact Profile – 68" test data.

The frequency of functional limitations according to the "Sickness Impact Profile – 68" test is shown in Fig. 2.

General assessment of the impact of the disease on the functional condition of patients is presented in Table 10 and Figure 3.

Table 10. Assessment (in points) of the disease impact on the functional condition of patients according to the "Sickness Impact Profile – 68" test data.

Behavior categories	Average point	Total point	Maximum possible point	% in relation to the maximum possible point
Social behavior	6.4±0.5	277	540	51
Degree of mobility	4.3±0.4	98	450	22
Psychic autonomy and communication	4±0.2	122	495	25
Mobility control	3.5±0.3	89	540	16
Emotional stability	3±0.2	70	270	26
Somatic autonomy	2.2±0.4	80	765	10

Thus, the patients with a diagnosis of acute disseminated encephalomyelitis showed functional condition impairment most often in the categories "social behavior", less frequently there were observed changes in the categories "somatic autonomy" and "psychic autonomy and communication." The categories "mobility control", "emotional stability," "degree of mobility" suffered the least frequently. The highest percent in relation to the maximum possible point was observed in the category "social behavior", and the lowest - in the category "somatic autonomy".

Assessment of the functional limitations of patients with ADEM according to the "Functional Limitation Profile" test data depending on gender and on the clinical course of ADEM.

Correlation analysis revealed a statistically significant direct relationship between the degree of functional limitations in patients with ADEM and age of the patients (correlation coefficient $r = 0.44$; $P < 0.001$), so the older the age is, the higher the degree of functional limitations caused by the emergence of the disease is. Thus, the age factor significantly affects the quality of life of patients with ADEM, as manifested by the presence of more pronounced limitations in the spheres of patients' life connected with the disease emergence. Statistical analysis of the results, obtained using the $\chi 2$ test, showed the relationship between gender and the degree of functional limitations in patients with ADEM. The results of survey of patients, diagnosed with acute disseminated encephalomyelitis according to the test "Functional Limitation Profile", that was confirmed statistically using Student's criteria for two independent selections, showed that compared to women men demonstrate greater changes associated with disease progression in category "social interaction" and "communication" (respectively 423.6 ± 9.5 points (men) and 263.8 ± 28.9 points (women), P <0.001 and 145.5 ± 2.8 points (men) and 82.6 ± 5.3 points (women), P <0.001).

Thus, the presence of the disease more affects the social activity of men. However, women perceive the presence of disease more emotionally (average indices of the changes in the category "emotion" are 81.5 ± 1.1 points (men) and 151 ± 9 points (women), P <0.001). Women also demonstrate more pronounced changes in the category "sleep and rest" (12 ± 5.9 points (men) and 128.6 ± 8.1 points (women), P <0.001) (Table 11).

Table 11. Assessment (in points) of the functional limitations of patients with ADEM according to the "Functional Limitation Profile" test data depending on gender.

Behavior categories	Men (n=20)	Women (n=25)
Social interaction	423.6±9.5	263.8±28.9*
Clarity of mind	338±31.8	257.2±24.2
Body care and motion	273±93	284.4±49.2
Household activity	255±37	217.4±29.6
Leisure and entertainments	194.5±28	184±10.9
Walk	179±40	213.7±21.7
Movement	171±18	188.7±18.5

Work	152.1±13.6	194.6±17
Communication	145.5±2.8	82.6±5.3*
Emotions	81.5±1.1	151±9*
Sleep and rest	12±5.9	128.6±8.1*
Food	34	34

Note. * – reliability of the difference of indices between groups of patients is P <0.001.

There is also a statistically significant relationship between the clinical course of disseminated encephalomyelitis (a first episode of acute encephalomyelitis or its multiphasic course) and the degree of functional limitation of patients ($\chi2$ - 374, P <0.001). The use of Student's test for two independent selections (tab. 12) also found differences in functional limitations according to the "Functional Limitation Profile" test in patients with a first episode of disseminated encephalomyelitis and its multiphasic course. Changes in emotional state associated with presence of the disease, were more pronounced in the patients with multiphasic course, compared to patients with a first episode of disseminated encephalomyelitis (243 points and 135.6 ± 7.6 points respectively, P <0.001). Patients with multiphasic course of disseminated encephalomyelitis, compared to patients with a first episode of its onset, had more pronounced changes in the category "sleep and rest" and less pronounced – in the category "communication" (122.3 ± 6.1 points (patients with a first episode of onset of disseminated encephalomyelitis) and 181.5 ± 40.4 points respectively (patients with multiphasic course of disseminated encephalomyelitis), P <0/01 and 104 ± 4.6 points (patients with a first episode of onset of disseminated encephalomyelitis) and 48.5 ± 0.7 points (patients with multiphasic course of disseminated encephalomyelitis), P <0.001).

Table 12. Assessment (in points) of the functional limitations of patients with ADEM according to the "Functional Limitation Profile" test data depending on the type of course of ADEM.

Behavior categories	A first episode of the demyelinating disease	Multiphasic course of disseminated encephalomyelitis
Social interaction	186.7±15.6	384.5±146.8
Clarity of mind	280.5±46.2	299.3±141
Body care and motion	170.8±12.7	333±119.9
Household activity	223.1±25.8	223.3±95
Leisure and entertainments	183.8±11.2	207.5±33.7

Walk	293.1±33.7	311.8±122.3
Movement	135.6±7.6	243*
Work	269.3±21.5	302.5±82.6
Communication	122.3±6.1	181.5±40.4^
Emotions	34	-
Sleep and rest	104±4.6	48.5±0.7*
Food	181±13.7	227.5±77.6

Note. * - The reliability of differences in results of the groups of patients with a first episode of demyelinating disease and with mulitiphasic course of disseminated encephalomyelitis is P <0.001, ^ - P <0.01.

Quality of life measures pursue the important goal of assessing the disease impact in patients' terms. In quality of life questionnaires the patient is invited to self-asses his/her life satisfaction (general or overall well-being), emotional or psychiatric symptoms such as anxiety or depression (cognitive component, evaluation of emotional feelings), symptoms of the disease (such as pain, fatigue etc.), and the functional impact of the disease (such as ability to ambulate, self-care, occupational performance, social and family participation, etc.)[47]. "Functional Limitation Profile" and "Sickness Impact Profile - 68" tests measures allow an understanding of the impact of ADEM on the patient's life, providing additional information to those obtained by the traditional objective clinical instruments of measurement of disease severity , such as, for example, the EDSS.

Despite the obvious importance of patients' self-assessment of their quality of life and assessment of impact of ADEM on their quality of life, this question has not been widely studied so far.

In our study the analysis of interrogation of patients with acute disseminated encephalomyelitis according to the tests "Functional Limitation Profile" and "Sickness Impact Profile - 68" showed significant changes of their functional condition connected with the occurrence of the disease.

The patients with a diagnosis of acute disseminated encephalomyelitis according to the test "Functional Limitation Profile" showed the impairment of functional condition most often in 3 categories: "work", "leisure and entertainment", "social interaction". Categories "communication", "emotion", "food" were the least impaired.

The patients with a diagnosis of acute disseminated encephalomyelitis according to the test "Sickness Impact Profile - 68" showed functional condition impairment most often in the categories "social behavior", the categories "mobility control", "emotional stability", "degree of mobility" were the least impaired. The highest percent in relation to the maximum possible point was observed in the category "social behavior", and the lowest - in the category "somatic autonomy".

For the more accurate assessment of the disease impact on the functional status of patients with ADEM it is advisable to compare this patients to a socio-demographically-matched healthy control group regarding their quality of life and assess the value of psychosocial functioning and quality of life measures as discrimination markers between patients with ADEM and healthy individuals.

Also for the most accurate assessment of the disease impact on the functional status of patients diagnosed with acute disseminated encephalomyelitis it is advisable to carry out their secondary interrogation depending on the transformation of ADEM into multiple sclerosis). Such interrogation of patients in the disease dynamics enables detecting possible changes in the categories of life that are the most affected by the disease occurrence. The perspective direction of the future studies is assessment of quality of life of patients with different variants of acute disseminated encephalomyelitis course aimed at discovering a possible retrospective link between the variant of the disease course and categories of life of patients that are impaired the most by the disease occurrence.

Therefore, according to the results of two tests ("Functional Limitation Profile" and "Sickness Impact Profile - 68"), the presence of acute disseminated encephalomyelitis significantly affects the quality of life of patients. It results in appearance of functional limitations in all spheres of life, most frequently – in the social sphere, least frequently – in the emotional sphere. Severity of neurologic deficit and increase in the number of demyelination foci on MRI have a negative impact on patients' self-assessment of their quality of life. However, gender of patients and the presence of disseminated encephalomyelitis relapses influence on the degree of functional limitation. The disease has a significant impact on the emotional state of women and patients with multiphasic course of disseminated encephalomyelitis. It is also reflected in the disorders of their sleep and rest. Social sphere of life is suffering more in men and patients with a first episode of disseminated encephalomyelitis.

Figure 1. The structure of functional limitations in patients with acute disseminated encephalomyelitis according to the "Functional Limitation Profile" test data.

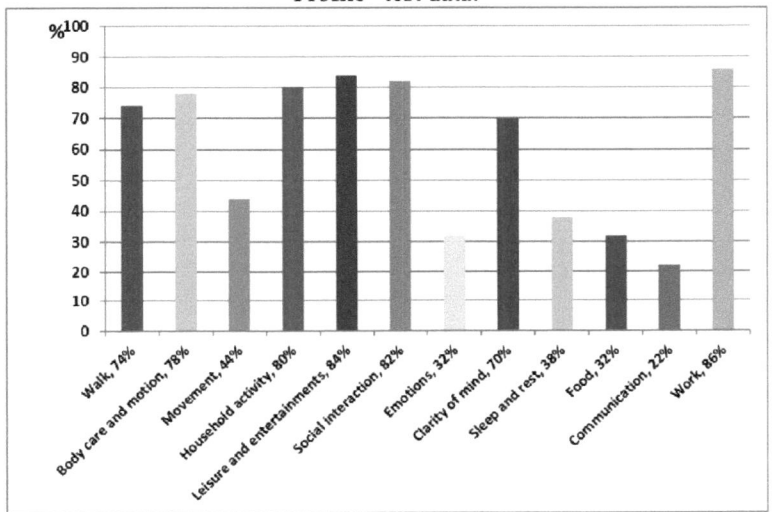

Figure 2. The structure of functional limitations in patients with acute disseminated encephalomyelitis according to the "Sickness Impact Profile – 68" test data.

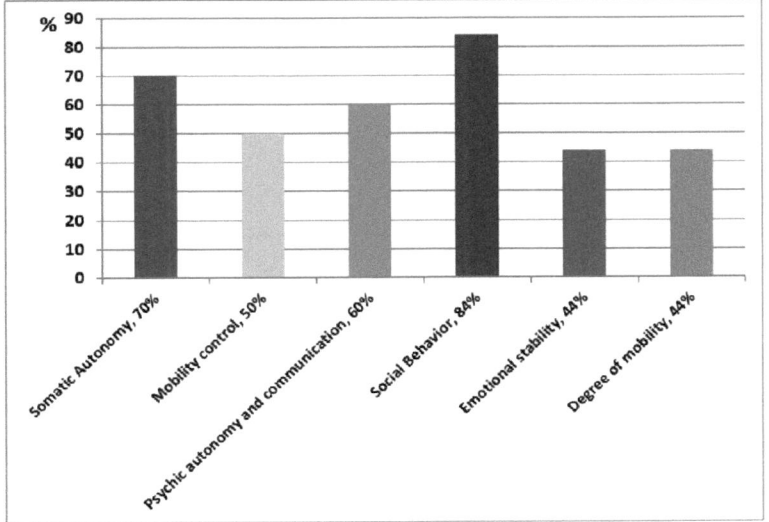

Figure 3. Assessment in points of functional limitations in patients with acute disseminated encephalomyelitis according to the "Sickness Impact Profile – 68" test data (% in relation to the maximum possible point).

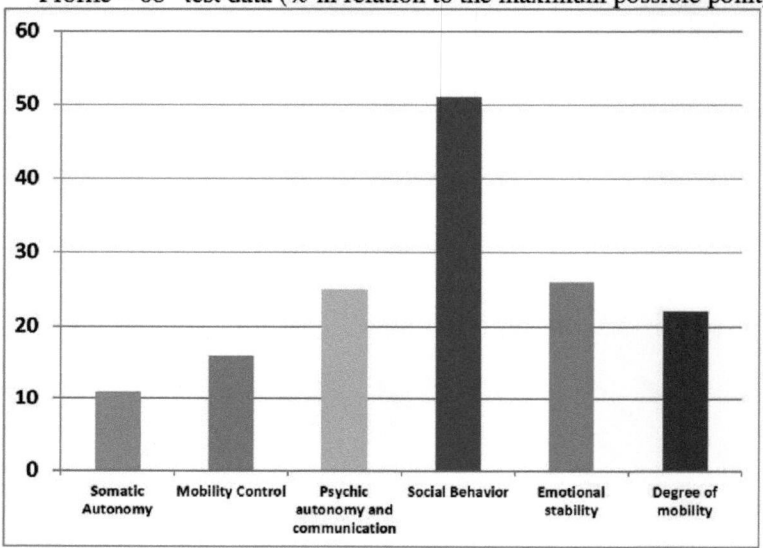

Prediction of multiphase alternative of acute disseminated encephalomyelitis course development.

To ascertain the prognostic meaning of clinic-paraclinic indices for patients with ADEM, we estimated the cumulative part of the absence of relapses by using the Kaplan-Meyer method with the Fisher criterion and the most important clinic-paraclinic data [97, 98].

The total prediction of cumulative parts for ADEM relapses in the form of its multi-phase course is adduced in Fig. 1.

As seen from Fig. 4, 10% (cumulative part is equal to 0.1) of patients with ADEM show the relapse 4 months after first signs of this disease, 25% (cumulative part – 0.25) –after the half-year (6 months), 50% (cumulative part – 0.5) –after one year (12 months), 75% (cumulative part – 0.75) –after 1.5 year (18 months) of the period for observation. The cumulative part of patients without relapses for the first 6 months was 0.75 (i.e., 75% of all the patients), for 12 months – 0.5 (50% of patients), for 24 months – 0.05 (5% of patients).

The dynamics of decay in the cumulative part of patients with ADEM but without relapses in the multiphase course within the three year period of observations is depicted in Fig. 5.

As seen in Fig. 2, in case of patients with the multiphase course of disseminated encephalomyelitis, the most pronounced decay in the cumulative part of patients without relapses was observed during the first year of observations (50%), somewhat less – during the second year (45%), and the least one – during the third year (5%).

Thus, the frequency of relapses changed in dependence on the term of observations for three year period, and it was the highest during the first year and the lowest during the third year.

The prognostic estimate of development inherent to the multiphase course of ADE in dependence on the age is depicted in Fig. 6.

As seen in Fig. 3, the best indices of replace absence were observed in patients of the age 39 to 40 years, however the statistical difference is not reliable ($p = 0.067$ (>0.05)).

Prediction of development of the multiphase course in ADEM in dependence on gender did not find any reliable difference between the three-year absence of replaces in men and women, but one could observe a tendency of increasing the cumulative part in women ($p = 0.07213$, (>0.05)) (Fig. 7).

Thus, one can draw a conclusion that such prognostic signs as age and gender have no reliable influence on development of relapses in ADEM in the form of its multiphase course.

Availability of changes in the neurologic status in the form of coordinative impairments is combined with development of MDEM in earlier terms of observation as compared with neurologic deficiencies in the form of motor impairments, which is an important prognostic sign ($p = 0.02803$, (<0.05)) (Fig. 8).

The complex estimate of the status of patients with ADEM by the EDSS scale and its relation with the term of appearance of MDEM signs are depicted in Fig. 9.

As seen in Fig. 6, the multiphase course of ADEM arose later (beginning from 9 months) in patients with a slight disability degree by the EDSS scale, as compared to those with a medium or heavy disability degrees ($p = 0.00141$, (< 0.001)).

Thus, availability of a slight disability degree by the above scale corresponds to a more positive course of ADEM, which is manifested in the increased cumulative part of patients without relapses as well as term of MDEM emergence.

When analyzing the MRT data taken from patients with ADEM, we ascertained that availability of demyelination focuses with various medium sizes makes an essential effect on prediction of the ADEM course, in particular its multiphase option, which is adduced in Fig. 10.

Thus, the smaller is the medium size of demyelination focuses, the slower is development of the multiphase course in this disease (replaces begin to arise after the first year of observations ($p = 0.02179$, (< 0.05)).

Thus, our analysis of the main clinic-paraclinic indices by the Kaplan-Meyer method proved to be reliable and enabled us to find out a number of important prognostic criteria of the multiphase course appearance in ADEM. The reliable influence on development of the multiphase course in ADEM is related to such prognostic signs as changes of the neurologic status in patients with ADEM, disability degree by the EDSS scale as well as size of demyelination focuses in accord with MRT data. The criteria for favorable prediction in this disease with later development of ADEM replaces in the form of multiphase course are domination of motor impairments over the coordination ones in the neurologic status, slight degree of disability by the EDSS scale, and small size (up to 4 mm) of demyelination focuses (MRT data).

Fig. 4. Dynamics of the cumulative part of patients with ADEM without development of the multiphase course for the three year period of observations (by the Kaplan-Meyer method).

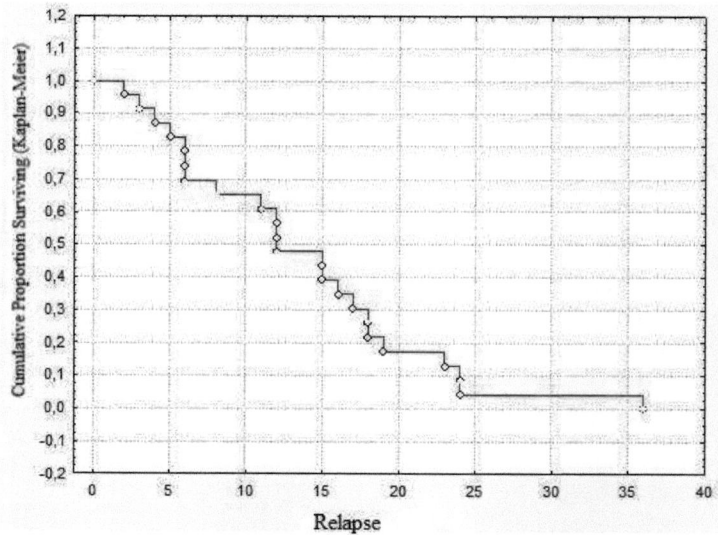

Fig. 5. Dynamics of decrease in the cumulative part of patients with ADEM but without development of the multiphase course in this disease for the three year period of observations (in %).

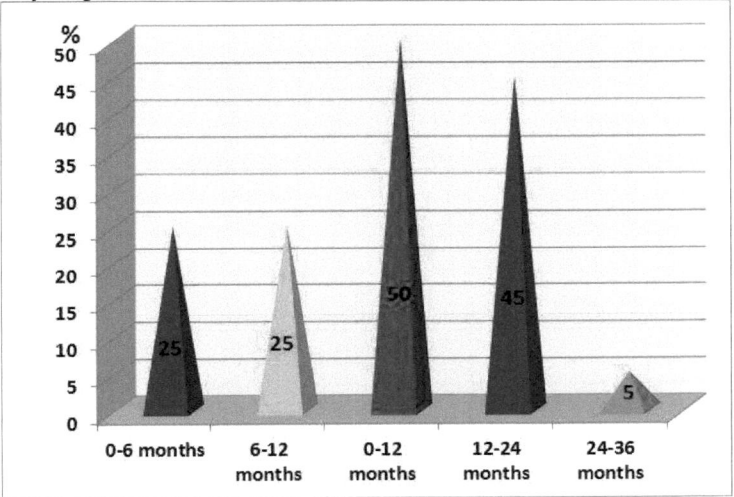

Fig. 6. Dynamics of the cumulative part of patients without relapses by separate age groups (using the Kaplan-Meyer method).

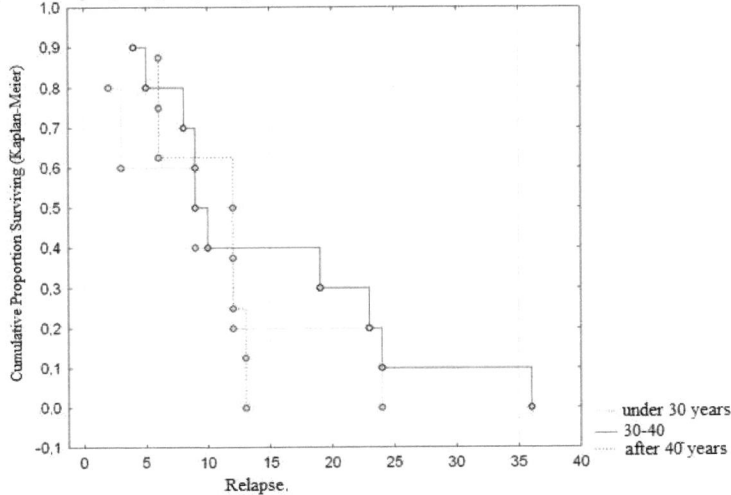

Fig. 7. Dynamics of the cumulative part of patients without relapses in dependence on their gender (by the Kaplan-Meyer method).

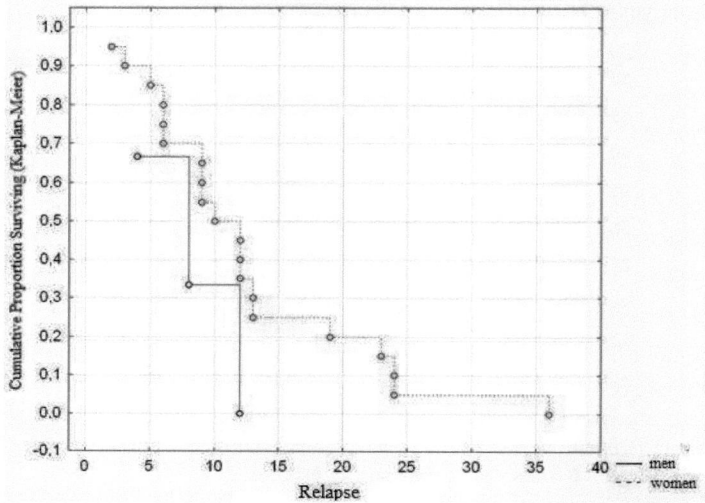

Fig. 8. Dynamics of the cumulative part of patients without relapses in dependence on changes in the neurologic status (by Kaplan-Meyer).

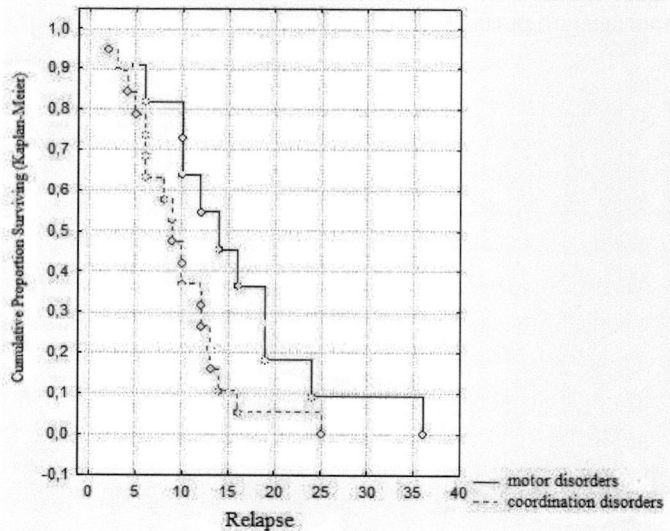

Fig. 9. Dynamics of the cumulative part of patients without relapses by the disability degree in accord with the EDSS scale (by Kaplan-Meyer).

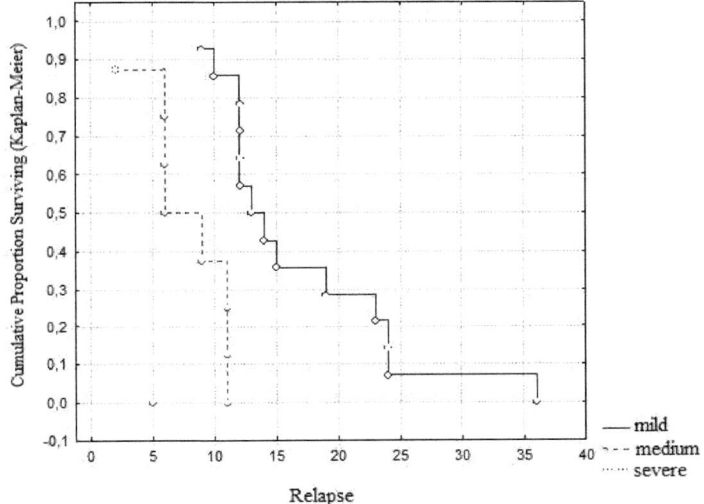

Fig. 10. Dynamics of the cumulative part of patients without relapses by sizes of demyelination focuses in accord with MRT data (by Kaplan-Meyer).

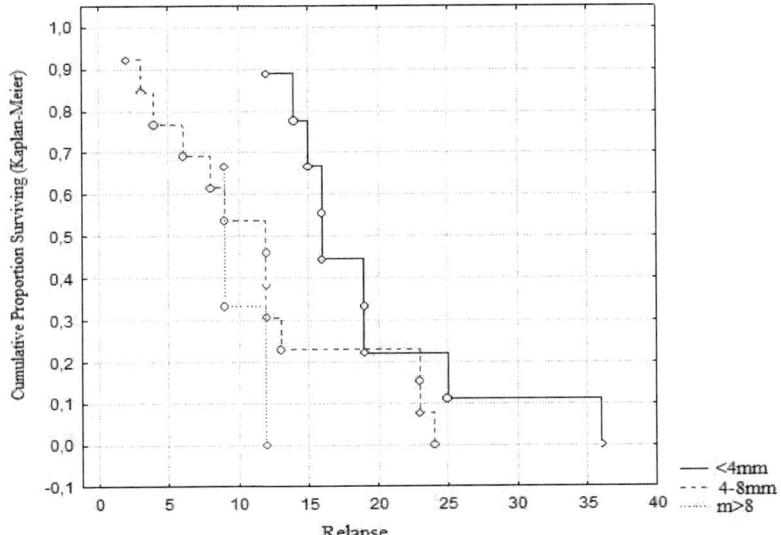

Prediction of transformation of acute disseminated encephalomyelitis into multiple sclerosis

To ascertain the prognostic meaning of clinic-paraclinic indexes for patients with ADEM, we estimated the cumulative part of the absence of relapses by using the Kaplan-Meyer method with the Fisher criterion and the most important clinic-paraclinic data [97, 98].

The total prediction of cumulative parts for transformation of ADEM into disseminated sclerosis is adduced in Fig. 11.

As seen from Fig. 1, 10% (cumulative part is equal to 0.1) of patients with ADEM show transformation of ADEM into multiple sclerosis 5 months after the first signs of this disease, 25% (cumulative part – 0.25) –after 7 months, 50% (cumulative part – 0.5) –after 11 months, 75% (cumulative part – 0.75) – after 15 months of the period for observation. The cumulative part of patients without transformation of ADEM into multiple sclerosis for the first 6 months was 0.78 (i.e., 78% of all the patients), for 12 months – 0.36 (36% of patients), for 24 months – 0.04 (4% of patients).

The dynamics of decay in the cumulative part of patients with ADEM but without replaces in its transformation into multiple sclerosis within the three year period of observations is depicted in Fig. 12.

As seen in Fig. 12, in case of patients with transformation of ADEM into multiple sclerosis, the most pronounced decay in the cumulative part of patients without relapses was observed during the first year of observations (64%) (in particular from 6 to 12 months (42%)), and the least pronounced – during the third year (4%).

Thus, the frequency of replaces changed in dependence on the term of observations for three year period, and it was the highest during the first year and the lowest during the third year.

The prognostic estimate of development for transformation of ADEM into multiple sclerosis in dependence on the age is depicted in Fig. 13.

As seen in Fig. 13, the best indices of relapses absence were observed in patients of the age 39 to 40 years, however the statistical difference is not reliable (p = 0,78019 (>0.05)).

Prediction of development of transformation of ADEM into multiple sclerosis in dependence on gender did not find any reliable difference between the three year absence of relapses in men and women, but one could observe a tendency for increasing the cumulative part in women (p = 0.15560 (>0.05)) (Fig. 14).

Thus, one can draw a conclusion that such prognostic signs as age and gender have no reliable influence on development of transformation of ADEM into multiple sclerosis.

The reliable difference for patients without replaces between the groups of patients with different changes in neurologic status was not found, in other words, presence of some neurologic deficiencies in patients with ADEM does not influence sufficiently on its transformation into multiple sclerosis.

The complex estimate of the status of patients with ADEM by the EDSS scale and its relation to the term of appearance of transformation of ADEM into multiple sclerosis are depicted in Fig. 15.

As seen in Fig. 16, transformation of ADEM into multiple sclerosis arose later in patients with a slight disability degree by the EDSS scale, as compared to those with a medium or heavy disability degrees; transformation of ADEM into multiple sclerosis arose later in patients with a heavy disability degree, but as far as after 25 months of observation multiple sclerosis arises in 100% of the patients of this group ($p = 0.01516$ (< 0.01)).

Thus, availability of a slight disability degree by the above scale corresponds to a more positive course of ADEM, which is manifested in prolongation of the term of emergence of ADEM transformation into multiple sclerosis.

When analyzing the MRT data taken from patients with ADEM, we ascertained that availability of demyelination focuses with various medium sizes makes an essential effect on prediction of the ADEM course, in particular its transformation into multiple sclerosis, which is adduced in Fig. 17.

Thus, the bigger is the medium size of demyelination focuses, the slower is development of transformation of ADEM into multiple sclerosis. ($p = 0.01757$ (< 0.05)).

Thus, our analysis of the main clinic-paraclinic indexes by the Kaplan-Meyer method proved to be reliable and enabled us to find out a number of important prognostic criteria of the ADEM course in the form of its transformation into multiple sclerosis. The reliable influence on development of transformation of ADEM into multiple sclerosis is related to such prognostic signs as disability degree by the EDSS scale and size of demyelination focuses in accord with MRT data. The most favorable criteria for prediction in this disease with later development of transformation into multiple sclerosis are slight degree of disability by the EDSS scale and large size of demyelination focuses (MRT data).

Fig. 11. Dynamics of the cumulative part of patients with ADEM without development of transformation of ADEM into multiple sclerosis for the three-year period of observations (by the Kaplan-Meyer method).

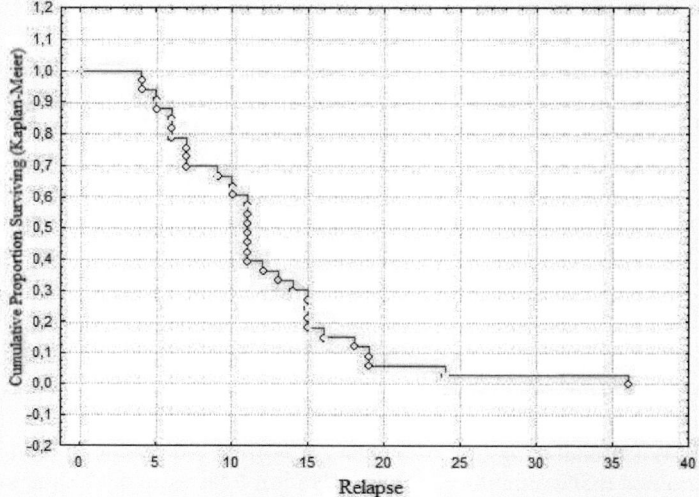

Fig. 12. Dynamics of decrease in the cumulative part of patients with ADEM but without development of transformation of ADEM into multiple sclerosis for the three year period of observations (in %).

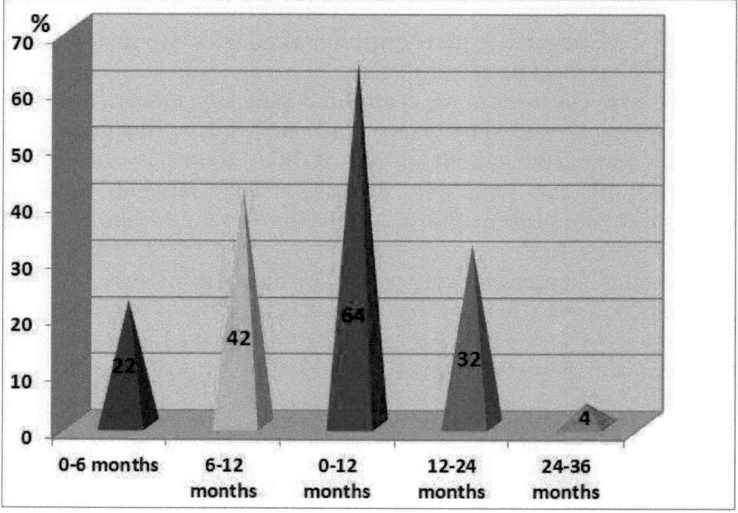

Fig. 13. Dynamics of the cumulative part of patients without replaces by separate age groups (using the Kaplan-Meyer method).

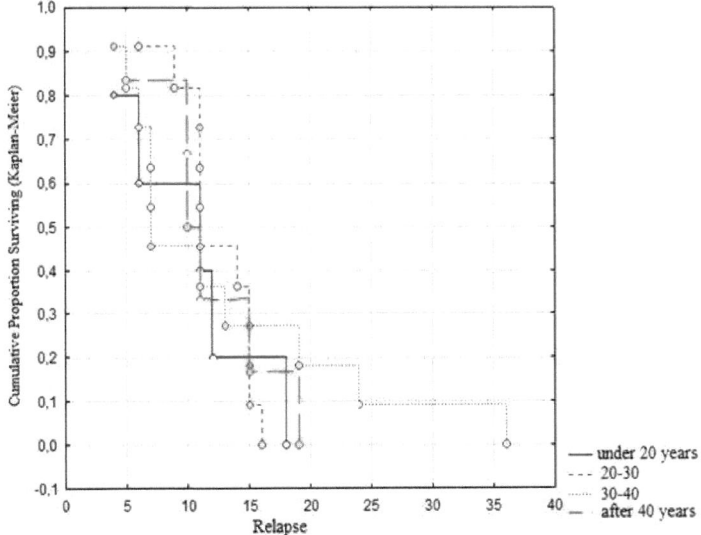

Fig. 14. Dynamics of the cumulative part of patients without replaces in dependence on their gender (by the Kaplan-Meyer method).

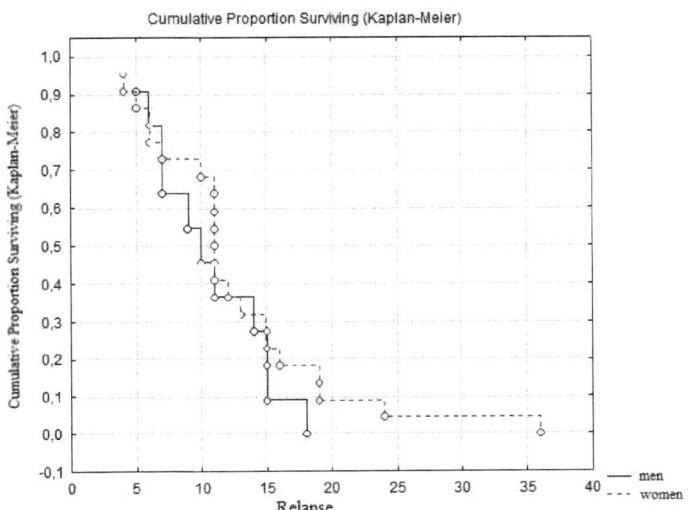

Fig. 15. Dynamics of the cumulative part of patients without relapses in dependence on changes in the neurologic status (by Kaplan-Meyer).

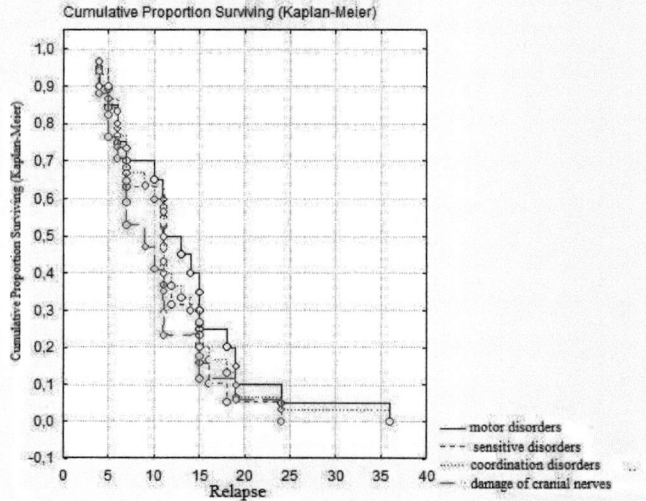

Fig. 16. Dynamics of the cumulative part of patients without relapses by the disability degree in accord with the EDSS scale (by Kaplan-Meyer).

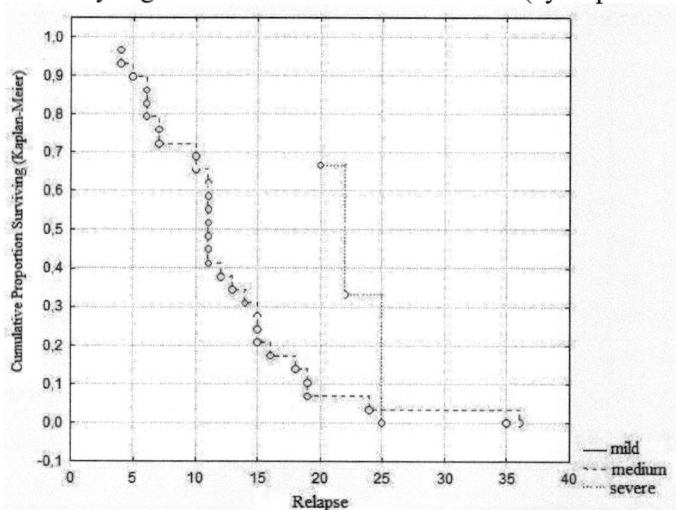

Fig. 17. Dynamics of the cumulative part of patients without relapses by sizes of demyelination focuses in accord with MRT data (by Kaplan-Meyer).

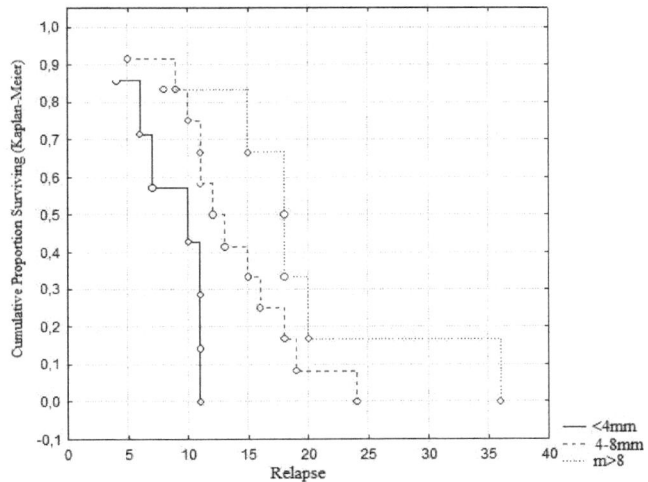

Analysis of prognostic significance of clinical and paraclinical indices in case of different types of acute disseminated encephalomyelitis course.

Statistical analysis of the results was made with the use of Stata 12. Generalized characteristic of the investigated indices is represented by the arithmetic mean (X). Variability of parameters was assessed by standard deviation. Change of parameters is presented in % with 95% confidence interval. For comparative analysis there was used t-test, chi-square test and Wilcoxon rank test [98].

According to the results of our research, during the 3-year period of observations there were noted the following variants were noted: 49 patients (48.5%) demonstrated monophasic variant of acute disseminated encephalomyelitis, 25 patients (24.8%) – multiphasic variant of its course, 27 patients (26.7%) noted the transformation of acute disseminated encephalomyelitis into multiple sclerosis (table. 13).

Table 13. Differentiation of patients with ADEM depending on the type of the course.

Type of the course	Number of patients	%
Monophasic	49	48,5

Multiphasic	25	24,8
Transformation into MS	27	26,7

Monophasic course of acute disseminated encephalomyelitis is more frequent than acute disseminated encephalomyelitis evolved to multiple sclerosis and multiphasic course of the disease.

The patients with MDEM had relapses in average $11,4 \pm 1,3$ months after the occurrence of the first episode of the disease. The patients with acute disseminated encephalomyelitis transformation into multiple sclerosis demonstrated development of multiple sclerosis on average after $12,04 \pm 1,75$ months. Demographic characteristic of patients with monophasic, multiphasic course of ADEM and ADEM transformation into multiple sclerosis is shown in Tables 14 and 15.

Table 14. Demographic characteristic of patients with monophasic course of ADEM and its transformation into multiple sclerosis

Index	Type of the course		p
	Monophasic	Transformation into multiple sclerosis	
Age (X±σ)	32.1±7.9	31.8±8.5	0.851*
Sex (n, %)			
Male	9 (18%)	11 (41%)	0,165**
Female	40 (82%)	16 (59%)	

* - t-test estimation;

** - chi-square test for independence groups.

Table 15. Demographic characteristic of patients with multiphasic course of ADEM and its transformation into multiple sclerosis

Index	Type of the course		p
	Multiphasic	Transformation into multiple sclerosis	
Age (X±σ)	30.1±7.5	31.8±8.5	0.829*
Sex (n, %)			
Male	8 (32%)	11 (41%)	0,263**
Female	17 (68%)	16 (59%)	

* - t-test estimation;

** - chi-square test for independence groups.

Thus, the study groups are comparable in sex and age composition.

Clinical presentation of monophasic, multiphasic course of ADEM and ADEM transformation into multiple sclerosis is shown in Table 16.

Table 16. Clinical presentation of monophasic, multiphasic course of ADEM and its transformation into multiple sclerosis

Index	Type of the course				
	Transformation into multiple sclerosis	Monophasic	p	Multiphasic	p
Prior infection	3 (11,1%)	9 (18%)	>0.05	5 (20,0%)	>0.05
Prior immunization	2 (7,4%)	5 (10,2%)	>0.05	3 (12,0%)	>0.05
Polysymptomatic presentation	19 (70,4%)	43 (87,8%)	>0.05	17 (68,0%)	>0.05
Monosymptomatic presentation	1(3,7%)	2 (4,1%)	>0.05	3 (12,0%)	>0.05
Motor disturbances	20 (74,1 %)	43 (87,7%)	>0.05	17 (68,0%)	>0.05
Numbness/abnormal sensation	11 (40,7%)	17 (34,7%)	>0.05	9 (36,0%)	>0.05
Brain stem symptoms	13 (48,1%)	17(34,7%)	>0.05	13 (52,0%)	>0.05
Unilateral optic neuritis	3 (11,1%)	5 (10,2%)	>0.05	3 (12,0%)	>0.05
Bilateral optic neuritis	1 (3,7%)	-	>0.05	-	>0.05
Cerebellar symptoms	14 (51,8%)	23(46,9%)	>0.05	15 (60%)	>0.05
Encefalitis	1 (3,7%)	5 (10,2%)	>0.05	2 (8,0%)	>0.05
Myelitis	1(3,7%)	3 (6,1%)	>0.05	1 (4,0%)	>0.05
Encephalopathy	25 (92,6%)	47 (95,9%)	>0.05	21 (84,4%)	>0.05
Seizures	2 (7,4%)	5 (10,2%)	>0.05	3 (12,0%)	>0.05

* - t-test estimation between groups of patients with transformation into multiple sclerosis and monophasic course and transformation into multiple sclerosis and multiphasic course of the disease.

There were no significant differences between clinical presentation of monophasic, multiphasic course of ADEM and ADEM that evolved to MS.

Comparative assessment of the changes of clinical and paraclinical indices in groups with different types of ADEM course is shown in Tables 16, 17, 18. Statistically significant difference is found for all indices during 1 year period between comparable periods (p <0.0001). However the direction of change of some parameters is different depending on the type of course. Thus, in the group with monophasic course number of demyelination foci decreased almost to 0 after 3 months of observation - 91.8% of patients with monophasic course of disseminated encephalomyelitis had 0 number of nidi and respectively 0 diameter of nidi size. Intensity of perifocal edema reduced and number of points according to EDSS scale also significantly decreased.

The group of patients with ADEM transformation into multiple sclerosis demonstrate statistically significant (p <0.0001) increase of demyelination foci number, but decrease of their diameter and intensity of perifocal edema. The intensity of neurological symptoms also significantly increases; it is reflected in the increase of number of points on EDSS scale.

Table 17. Comparative characteristic of groups with monophasic type of ADEM course and its transformation into multiple sclerosis (X±σ)

Index	Type of course					
	Monophasic		p	Transformation into multiple sclerosis		p
	Period 0	Period 1		Period 0	Period 1	
Number of points according to EDSS scale	2.5±0.5	0.7±0.35	<0,0001	2.6±0.4	4.4±0.59	<0,0001
Number of demyelination foci	8.4±1.7	0.1±0.3	<0,0001	10.3±2.9	13.2±2.7	<0,0001
Diameter of demyelination foci	9.5±0.9	0.35±1.2	<0,0001	9.1±0.7	4.9±1.6	<0,0001
Perifocal edema	10.0±2.1	0.16±0.56	<0,0001	9.7±2	3.5±2.1	<0,0001

p - Wilcoxon rank test estimation.

The main characteristics that create statistically significant difference for the monophasic type of ADEM course and its transformation into multiple sclerosis are reduction of the number of demyelination foci (-99.03%) and the number of points according to EDSS scale in case of monophasic course (-73.1%), but worsening (increase) of these indices in case of ADEM transformation into multiple sclerosis (respectively 32.6% and 71.9%). Thus, the nature of the changes of demyelination foci and the number of points according to EDSS scale are prognostically significant characteristics for assessment of monophasic course of ADEM and its transformation into multiple sclerosis (Table 18).

Table 18. The changes of clinical and paraclinical indices in groups with monophasic type of ADEM course and its transformation into multiple sclerosis
(Δ - % (95% CI))

| Index | Type of the course | | p |
	Monophasic	Transformation into multiple sclerosis	
Number of points according to EDSS scale,Δ,% (95%CI)	-73.1 (-75.3 – -70.8)	+71.9 (65.3 – 78.4)	<0,0001
Number of demyelination foci, Δ,%(95%CI)	-99.03 (-100 – -98.04)	+32.6 (27.5 – 37.7)	<0,0001
Diameter of demyelination foci, Δ,%(95%CI)	-95.93 (-99.9 – -91.9)	-45.5 (-50.8 – -40.1)	<0,0001
Perifocal edema, Δ,% (95%CI)	-98.2 (-100.0 – -96.3)	-62.4 (-69.2 – -55.6)	<0,0001

p – t-test estimation, CI – confidential interval, Δ - change of the index in %.

Table 19. Analysis of clinical and paraclinical parameters in group of patients with multiphasic type of ADEM and its transformation into multiple sclerosis ($X\pm\sigma$).

| Index | Type of the course | | | | | |
| | Multiphasic | | | Transformation into multiple sclerosis | | |
	Period 0	Period 1	p	Period 0	Period 1	p
Number of points	2.6±0.41	4.8±0.5	<0.001	2.6±0.4	4.4±0.59	<0.001

accor-ding to EDSS scale						
Number of demyli-nation foci	9.8±3.1	12±2.7	<0.001	10.±2.9	13.2±2.7	<0.001
Diameter of demyeli-nation foci	9.2±0.7	6.0±1.5	<0.001	9.1±0.7	4.9±1.6	<0.001
Perifocal edema	9.7±1.9	5.5±0.6	<0.001	9.7±2	3.5±2.1	<0.001

p - Wilcoxon rank test estimation.

Statistically significant difference between the studied indices of patients with ADEM in different periods of observation is detected both in case of multiphasic course of the disease and its transformation into multiple sclerosis.

Table 20. The changes of clinical and paraclinical indices in groups with multiphasic type of ADEM course and its transformation into multiple sclerosis
(Δ - % (95%CI))

| Index | Type of the course | | p |
	Multiphasic	Transformation into multiple sclerosis	
Dymanics of number of points according to EDSS scale, %	+85.4 (76.2 – 94.7)	+71.9 (65.3 – 78.4)	<0,0001
Dymanics of number of demyelination foci, %	+31.8 (24.5 – 39.1)	+32.6 (27.5 – 37.7)	0,742
Dymanics of diameter of	-33.6 (-41.9 – -25.3)	-45.5 (-50.8 – -40.1)	<0,0001

40

demyelination foci, %			
Dymanics of perifocal edema, %	-40.6 (-46.5 – (-34.7))	-62.4 (-69.2 – -55.6)	<0,0001

p – t-test estimation, CI – confidential interval, Δ - change of the index in %.

Increase of the number of demyelination foci in case of multiphasic course (31.8%) and in patients with ADEM transformation into multiple sclerosis (32.6%) does not differ statistically. For other indices there is observed statistically significant difference in their changes during the period of observation.. In case of multiphasic course (compared to the transformation into multiple sclerosis) reduction of the diameter of demyelination foci and perifocal edema is less pronounced, but increase of points according to EDSS scale is more intense (p <0.0001).

All the investigated clinical indices (number of points according to EDSS scale, number of foci of demyelination and their diameter, the presence of perifocal edema) and its changes during the period of observation are prognostically important for assessing the type of ADEM course (monophasic and transformation into multiple sclerosis). The given parameters (except changes of demyelination foci) significantly differ in case of multiphasic course of ADEM and its transformation into multiple sclerosis that proves their diagnostic value.

In case of monophasic type of ADEM course during a short period of time (up to 3 months) there was observed decrease of number of points according to EDSS scale, decrease of number and diameter of demyelination nidi (up to their almost complete reduction in 91.8% of patients), and decrease of perifocal edema.

In case of multiphasic type of ADEM course and in case of its transformation into multiple sclerosis, there was observed increase in the number of points according to EDSS scale and increase of number of demyelination nidi, but reduction of their diameter and perifocal edema, more pronounced in the case of transformation of ADEM into MS.

The major limitation of our work was that the study design was retrospective, so it does not allow a correct identification of prognostic factors.

Further studies should be aimed at determination of the prognostic significance of different methods of treatment of acute disseminated encephalomyelitis (therapy with corticosteroids, antiviral therapy) for prediction of different types of ADEM course.

When assessing the possible course of ADEM it is necessary to pay special attention to the clinical-paraclinical indices (number of points according to EDSS scale, number of foci of demyelination and their diameter, the presence of perifocal edema on MRI) in the process of dynamic observation. The changes of these indices has great value for prediction of monophasic, multiphasic types of ADEM course and its transformation into MS.

The efficacy of intravenous immunoglobulin in the treatment of patients with acute disseminated encephalomyelitis

Therapeutic efficacy of intravenous immunoglobulin was prospectively analyzed in the treatment of 27 patients with ADEM: 12 men and 15 women aged 17 – 53 (average index 31.7±1.6). Influence of the treatment on changes in neurological status of patients as well as variations in the disease course were studied.

10 patients with ADEM (21%) – 6 patients of the main group (22%) and 4 patients of the control group (20%) have the medical history of preceding signs of infectious process. The onset of disease in all patients was acute with evident disseminated lesion of central nervous system, frequently involving gray matter of the brain, increase of neurological deficit was observed during the short period of time (hours – days) and sudden development of encephalopathy.

The patients were randomly separated into two groups depending on the treatment method. All patients were blinded to their treatment group. According to indications the treatment in both main and control group was preceded by premedication with hormonal pulse-therapy, using methylprednisolone in the dose of 500-1000 mg daily in 200 ml of isotonic sodium chloride solution (within 5 days). The first (main) group included 27 patients who were daily administrated intravenous immunoglobulin in the dose of 0.4 g per 1 kg of mass of body within 5 days 1 month after the hormonal pulse-therapy. The treatment was followed by monthly administration of human normal immunoglobulin – 0.4 g per 1 kg of body mass within 24 months as a method of ADEM monotherapy. The control group included 20 patients aged 19 – 51 (average index 36 ± 3) with the same demographic characteristics. Intravenous administration of human normal immunoglobulin was not used in the treatment of control group patients. The participants of this group were given placebo treatment (200 ml of isotonic sodium chloride solution).

All the patients were under observation by the same physicians for 24 months. In case of the disease relapses, the patients of both main and control group received the same hormonal pulse-therapy, using methylprednisolone in the dose of 500-1000 mg daily in 200 ml of isotonic sodium chloride solution (within 5 days).

Therapeutic efficacy of the performed treatment of patients with ADEM was assessed by the amount of restored neurological functions (in points), using the Kurztke – Expanded Disability Status Score (EDSS) scale [90] and by the number of demyelination disease relapses over a 12-month period of observation. The decrease of neurological disorders index by 1.5-2 points according to EDSS scale was considered a significant improvement, the decrease by 1 point – a moderate improvement, the decrease by 0.5 point – an insignificant one. The absence of restored neurological functions according to the EDSS scale was assessed as an absence of therapeutic effect.

All the patients were under observation for 2 years. If during this period (2 years) no relapse of demyelination disease was detected, it was interpreted it as the monophasic type of the ADEM course. In the case when disease relapses appeared, having the signs of disseminated encephalomyelitis from the clinical viewpoint and after neuro-visual patient examination, it was considered as the multiphasic option of the disease course. In the case of clinically confirmed multiple sclerosis (in accord with the McDonald criteria [50]), we interpreted it as transition of ADEM into multiple sclerosis.

Statistical analysis of the results was made with the use of Stata 12. Generalized characteristic of the investigated indices is represented by the arithmetic mean (X). Variability of parameters was assessed by standard deviation. For comparative analysis there was used t-test (five percent for two tailed tests was chosen as the level of significance) and χ^2 test ($\alpha=0.05$, two sided). The Fisher criterion was used for two-group comparisons of frequency of relapses over a 24-month observation period.

Demographic data are shown in Table 21.

Table 21. Demographic and clinical profile of participants

Variable	Main group	Control group	P value
Overall numbers (%)	27	20	-
Baseline age, years	31.7±1.6	31.9±1.5	0.2
Gender			
Male	12 (40%)	7 (35%)	0.6
Female	15 (60%)	13 (65%)	0.6
Race			
White	27 (100%)	20 (100%)	-

Disability level according to the EDSS scale, points			
Overall score	3.8±0.2	3.9±0.2	0.7
Mild (1.0-3.5)	n = 16 (3 ± 0.1)	n = 12 (3.1 ± 0.1)	0.5
Moderate (4.0-6.0)	n = 10 (4.8±0.2)	n = 8 (4.3±0.2)	0.4
Severe (6.5-9.0)	n = 1 (6.5)	-	-

Note. Average index of the points according to the EDSS scale is given in brackets.

The analysis of pre-treatment clinical and neurological examination data shows that disability level at baseline (in points) was the same in both clinical groups (Table 21). The disability of patients according to the EDSS scale mostly had mild and moderate level, much less frequently – severe one.

CSF was analyzed in all 47 patients (both main and control group). CSF evidence of inflammation (either pleocytosis or elevated protein) was present in 39 patients (82,9%). The CSF White Blood Cells (WBC) count ranged between 0 and 137 with a mean of 40,8 cells/mm3. WBC count was elevated in 17 patients (25,5%). The CSF protein ranged between 0.33 mmol/L and 0.9 mmol/L with a mean of 0.6mmol/L.The CSF protein elevated in 32 patients (68.1%). CSF glucose concentrations were normal in all patients. Oligoclonal IgG bands *in* cerebrospinal fluid were not detected.

The use of immunomodulating method – human normal immunoglobulin for intravenous administration – in the treatment of the patients with ADEM had the positive influence on restoring the neurological functions and reducing the disability level in the EDSS points. It has been confirmed by the results of therapy of patients of the main and control groups (their average disability indices are given in Table 22 and Fig. 18).

Table 22. Changes of average index of EDSS functional system in patients with ADEM of different clinical groups.

Functional systems	Clinical group of patients with ADEM	Disability level according to the EDSS **functional system**, points	
		Before treatment	1 month after beginning of the treatment
Impairment of pyramidal tract	main	4.5±0.3	3,1±0.3*
	control	4.1±0.3	3.5±0.3

Impairment in coordination sphere	main	3.5±0.3	2,7±0.3*
	control	3.6±0.3	3,1±0.3
Urine bladder disorders	main	2,1±0.3	1.8±0.1
	control	2,3±0.3	2.1±0.1

Note. *– t-test estimation, reliability of difference between the indices before and after the treatment, p<0.05.

The results of neurological examination of patients over a 24-month period are shown in Table 23 and Fig. 19. One month after beginning of the treatment patients of both groups demonstrated the decrease of neurological deficit, measured according to the EDSS scale, compared to the indices before treatment (p<0.01). The patients of the main group showed a slight decrease of neurological deficit 12 months after leaving the hospital (p>0.05); the patients of the control group on the contrary showed the increase of neurologic deficit, yet not confirmed statistically (p>0.05). During the second examination after 12 months (24 months after beginning of the treatment) even more significant reduction of the level of neurological disorders of the patients of the main group (p<0.05) and its increase in the patients of the control group (p<0.05) was observed, which is explained by development of demyelination disease relapses over a 24-month observation period.

Table 23. Dynamics of changes in neurological status of patients with ADEM over a 24-month observation period.

Group of patients	Disability level according to the EDSS scale, points			
	Before treatment	1 month after beginning of the treatment	After 12 months	After 24 months
main (n=27)	3.8±0.2	3.0±0.2	2.8±0.3	2.3±0.4
control (n=20)	3.9±0.2	3.4±0.2	3.8±0.3*°	4.1±0.3°

Note. *– t-test estimation, p<0.05; ^ – p<0.001.
   ° - chi-square test for independence groups.

As can be seen from the Table 3, six and twelve months after beginning of the treatment, the patients of the control group demonstrated the increase of neurological deficit compared to the patients of the main group. Over a 24-month observation period, patients of both groups had on average 9 relapses, thus demonstrating multiphasic course of the disease. The patients of the main group had 2 relapses of disseminated encephalomyelitis and the patients of the control group had 7 relapses (multiphasic course of

ADEM). One woman from the control group had two relapses of disseminated encephalomyelitis over the year. Two patients from the control group demonstrated transformation of ADEM into MS, but they were discarded from the analysis. The frequency of demyelinating disease relapses was much lower in the patients of the main group (p<0,001) (Table 24).

Table 24. Frequency of relapses in the patients with ADEM over a 24-month observation period.

Clinical group of patients with ADEM	Observation period					
	1 month	6 months	12 months	18 months	24 months	Total number of relapses
main (n=27)	–	1	1	–	–	2 (7,4%)
control (n=20)	–	1	2	2	2	7 (35%) *°

Note. * - Fisher criterion, p<0.001.
 ° - chi-square test for independent groups.

Fig. 18. Dynamics of restoring neurological functions of patients with ADEM in different clinical groups as a result of treatment.

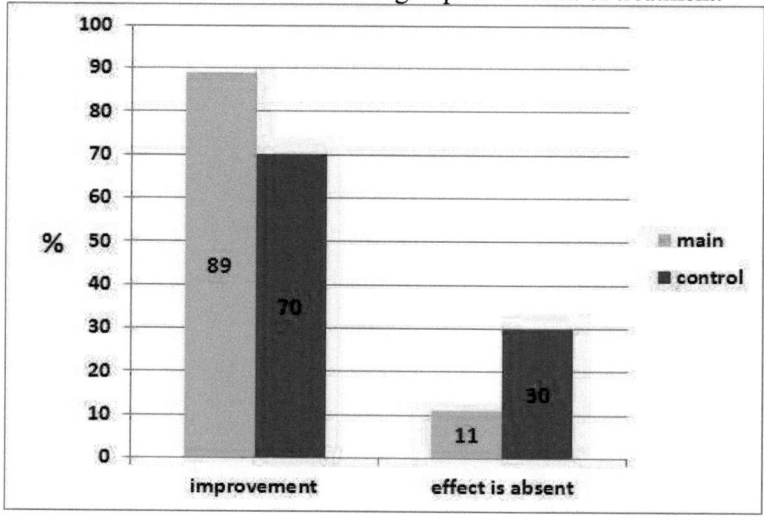

46

Fig. 19. Dynamics of changes in neurological status of patients with ADEM according to the EDSS scale over a 24-month observation period.

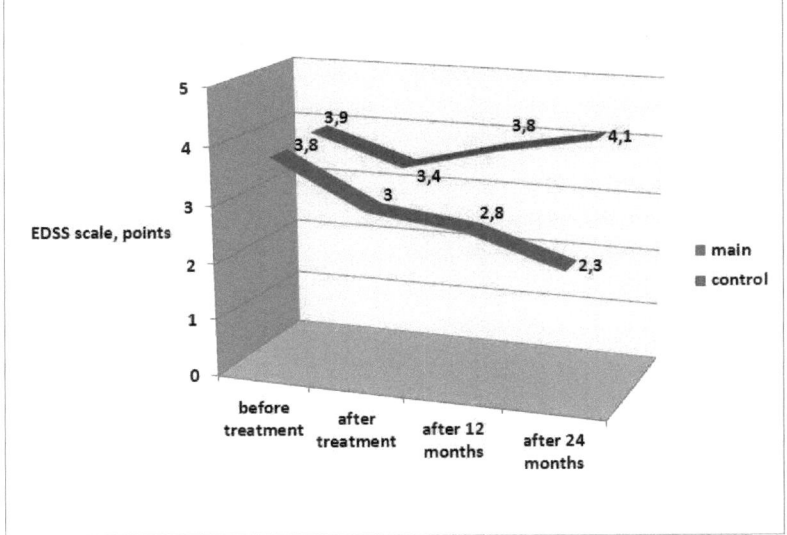

The performed investigations prove the positive therapeutic efficacy of intravenous administration of human normal immunoglobulin in the treatment of patients with acute disseminated encephalomyelitis.

Immunobiological action of immunoglobulin is believed to contribute to treatment efficacy due to the presence of antibodies against various infectious agents (virus of measles, influenza, varicella, parotitis, poliomyelitis, rubella, herpes-associated roup, hepatitis A and B, pneumococcus) [43, 98-109]. Its efficacy has been demonstrated in several controlled studies [106]. A broad spectrum of immunological mechanisms is thought to be relevant in explaining the properties of IV Ig therapy, such as supply of idiotypic antibodies, neutralization of complement-mediated effects [109], inhibition of complement binding and prevention of membranolytic attack complex (MAC), modulation of Fc receptos or T-cell function. In the treatment of neurological autoimmune disorders, only a few of these mechanisms seem to be relevant like the modulation of complement activation and activation and activity of macrophages [43, 109]. Experimental data show that in case of inflammatory diseases immunoglobulin may influence on the local immune response in the central nervous system, regulating nitric oxide release and microglia function [43,

110]. Remyelination stimulation can be a possible consequence of immunoglobulin use [43, 110, 111].

The use of intravenous immunoglobulin (IVIG) has been reported in several case studies as well, either alone [43, 112] or in combination with corticosteroids [43, 113]. There is a lack of specific recommendations for the long-term management of recurrent and multiphasic ADEM [114]. But several studies have reported a reduction of relapses after the long-term administration (every 4 weeks for 48 weeks) of intravenous immunoglobulin to patients with relapsing-remitting multiple sclerosis [114]. The results of the studies [43] has shown more significant reduction of the level of neurological disorders of the patients who received intravenous immunoglobulin in the dose of 0.4 g per 1 kg of mass of body within 5 days 1 month after the hormonal pulse-therapy, using methylprednisolone in the dose of 500-1000 mg daily in 200 ml of isotonic sodium chloride solution (within 5 days), comparing to the patients with placebo treatment (200 ml of isotonic sodium chloride solution) after the hormonal pulse-therapy. Over a 24-month observation period, the patients of the main group (who received intravenous immunoglobulin in the dose of 0.4 g per 1 kg of mass of body within 5 days 1 month after the hormonal pulse-therapy) had fewer relapses of disseminated encephalomyelitis comparing to the patients with placebo treatment. The results of the other studies and this case report proved that immunoglobulin administration contributes not only to the reduction of clinical manifestations of the disease by decreasing the level of neurologic deficit but also helps to prevent the disease relapses.

Conclusions:

Analysis of the obtained results showed that patients with ADEM had significantly lower cognitive scores of cognitive functions such as short and long term visual and auditory memory, verbal learning and delayed recall, sustained attention and concentration as well as memory, attention and orientation in time and space. The sequelae of cognitive disorders include negative impact on daily life activities, employment, social functioning and relations. Therapeutic correction of cognitive disorders in case of carrying out treatment-rehabilitation measures in patients with acute disseminated encephalomyelitis will improve the quality of life of patients.

According to the results of two tests ("Functional Limitation Profile" and "Sickness Impact Profile - 68"), the presence of acute disseminated encephalomyelitis significantly affects the quality of life of patients. It results in appearance of functional limitations in all spheres of life, most frequently – in the social sphere, least frequently – in the emotional sphere. The disease has a significant impact on the emotional state of women and patients with multiphasic course of disseminated encephalomyelitis. It is also reflected in the disorders of their sleep and rest. Social sphere of life is suffering more in men and patients with a first episode of disseminated encephalomyelitis.

The analysis of the main clinic-paraclinic indices by the Kaplan-Meyer method proved to be reliable and enabled us to find out a number of important prognostic criteria of the multiphase course appearance in ADEM. The reliable influence on development of the multiphase course in ADEM is related to such prognostic signs as changes of the neurologic status in patients with ADEM, disability degree by the EDSS scale as well as size of demyelination focuses in accord with MRT data. The criteria for favorable prediction in this disease with later development of ADEM replaces in the form of multiphase course are domination of motor impairments over the coordination ones in the neurologic status, slight degree of disability by the EDSS scale, and small size (up to 4 mm) of demyelination focuses (MRT data).

The reliable influence on development of transformation of ADEM into multiple sclerosis is related to such prognostic signs as disability degree by the EDSS scale and size of demyelination focuses in accord with MRT data. The most favorable criteria for prediction in this disease with later development of transformation into multiple sclerosis are slight degree of disability by the EDSS scale and large size of demyelination focuses (MRT data).

When assessing the possible course of ADEM it is necessary to pay special attention to the clinical-paraclinical indices (number of points according to EDSS scale, number of foci of demyelination and their diameter, the presence of perifocal edema on MRI) in the process of dynamic observation. The changes of these indices has great value for prediction of monophasic, multiphasic types of ADEM course and its transformation into MS.

This case report confirms a positive therapeutic efficacy of intravenous immunoglobulin in the treatment of patient with ADEM – reduction of clinical manifestations of the disease, in particular a decrease in neurological deficit level. Monthly intravenous immunoglobulin administration helps to prevent the disease relapses (multiphase ADEM course).

The results of our investigation proved a positive therapeutic efficacy of intravenous immunoglobulin in the treatment of patient with ADEM – reduction of clinical manifestations of the disease, in particular a decrease in neurological deficit level. Monthly intravenous immunoglobulin administration helps to prevent the disease relapses (multiphase ADEM course). According to the results of our study, monthly administration of human normal immunoglobulin is also of great prognostic importance for prevention of the multiphasic course of acute disseminated encephalomyelitis.

References:

1. Alexander M. , Murphy J. M. **Acute disseminated encephalomyelitis*; an update Arch Neural* (2011), 62(11):** 1673- 1680
2. Bergner M, Bobbit R, Carter W, Gilson B. The Sickness Impact Profile: **Development and Final Revision of a Health Condition Measure.** Med Care. 1981, 8:787-805.
3. Fridinger S.E, Alper G. **Severe Acute Disseminated Encephalomyelitis With Clinical Findings of Transverse Myelitis After Herpes Simplex Virus Infection.** *J Child Neurol,* 2014, **29:** 1519-1523.
4. Harris C. C. Harris, K. Lee J. **Acute disseminated encephalomyelitis.** *Neurosci. Nurs. –* 2007. **39 (4).** – P. 208 – 212.
5. Hasim HZ., Ibrahim N M. , Wanyahua N., Tan H J., et al. **A case of biopsy proven of acute disseminated encephalomyelitis with haemorrhagic lecoencephalitis.** *Ann Acad Med Singarope* (2011), **40(4):** 197-200.
6. Hoche F., Pfeifenbring S., Vlaho S., et al. **Rare brain biopsy findings in a first acute disseminated encephalomyelitis- like event of pediatric M. S.: histopathologic, neuroradiologic and clinical features** . *J. Neural Transm.* 2011, **118(9):** 1311-1317.
7. Lobanova I. **The Characteristics of Cognitive Functions in Patients with Acute Disseminated Encephalomyelitis.** *International Neuropsychiatric Disease Journal,* 2015, **3 (4):** 141-149.
8. Chowdhary J. **Measles with Acute Disseminated Encephalomyelitis (ADEM).** *Indian Pediatrics.* 2009, **46.**
9. Ogava Y. **A case of acute disseminated encephalomyelitis presenting with vertigo.** *Auris Nasus Larynx.* 2008, **35:** 127 – 130.
10. Sawanyawisuth K. **MRI findings in acute disseminated encephalomyelitis following varicella infection in an adult Case Reports.** *J. Clinical Neuroscience.* 2007, **14:** 1230 – 1233.
11. Voudris K.A. **Acute disseminated encephalomyelitis associated with parainfluenza virus infection of childhood.** *Brain Dev.* 2002, **24 (2):** 112 – 124.

12. Dale R.C. **Early relapse risk after a first CNS inflammatory demyelination episode: examining international consensus definitions.** *Dev. Med. Child Neurol.* 2007, **49 (12):** 887 – 893.

13. Kinomoto K. **Acute Encephalomyelitis Associated with Acute Viral Hepatitis Type B.** *Inter. Med.* 2009, **48**: 241 – 243.

14. Cahnzos-Romero T. **Demyelinating disorders: not only multiple sclerosis.** *Abstracts from 8th congress of the European Federation of Intern. Medicine.* 2009, **20:** 282 – 283.

15. Gard R.K. **Acute disseminated encephalomyelitis.** *Postgraduate Medical Journal.* 2003, **79**:11 – 17.

16. John W. Young. **Acute inflammatory encephalomyelitis following Campylobacter enteritis associated with high titre antiganglioside GM1 IgG antibodies Case Reports** *J. Clinical Neuroscience.* 2009, **16:** 597 – 598.

17. Njeukui T.J. **Acute disseminated encephalomyelitis associated with mycoplasma pneumoniaeinfection.** *Rev. Med. Brux.* 2008, **29 (2):** 103 – 106.

18. Stam B. **Neuroinvasion by Mycoplasma Pneumoniae in ADEM.** *International Journal of STG and AIDS.* 2006, **17 (7):** 493 – 495.

19. Stam B. **Neuroinvasion by Mycoplasma pneumoniae in acute disseminated encephalomyelitis.** *Emerg Infect Dis.* 2008, **14 (4):** 641 – 643.

20. Termote B. **Encephalitis following Mycoplasma pneumonia (2007: 6b). Acute disseminatedencephalomyelitis.** *Eur. Radiol.* 2007, **17 (9):** 2436 – 2438.

21. Gaing C. **Acute disseminated encephalomyelitis associated with Campylobacter jejuni infection and antiganglioside GM1 Ig G antibodies.** *J. Neurol.* 2005, **252**: 613 – 614.

22. Omata T. **Child with acute disseminated encephalomyelitis (ADEM) initially presenting with psychiatric symptoms.** *No To Hattatsu.* 2008, **40 (6):** 465 – 468.

23. Orr D. **Acute disseminated encephalomyelitis temporally associated with Campylobactergastroenteritis.** *J. Neurol. Neurosurg. Psychiatry.* 2004, **75 (5):** 792 – 793.

24. Murthy J. M. **Acute disseminated encephalomyelitis.** *Neurol.* 2002, **50**: 238 – 243.

25. Dale R.C. **Acute disseminated encephalomyelitis, multiphasic disseminated encephalomyelitis and multiple sclerosis in children** *Brain.* 2000, **123**: 2407 – 2224.

26. Gard R.K. **Acute disseminated encephalomyelitis.** *Postgraduate Medical Journal.* 2003, **79**: 11 – 17.

27. Ito S. **Acute disseminated encephalomyelitis and poststreptococcal acute glomerulonephritis.** *Brain Dev.* 2002, **24 (2):** 88 – 90.
28. Noel S. **Adult acute disseminated encephalomyelitis associated with poststreptococcalinfection.** *J. Clin. Neurosci.* 2005, **12 (3):** 298 – 300.
29. Fujikiet F. **Aseptic meningitis as initial presentation of ADEM** *.J. Neurol. Sci.* 2008, **272:** 129 – 131.
30. Samile N. **Acute disseminated encephalomyelitis in children. A descriptive study in Tehran, Iran.** *Saudi Med J.* 2007, **28 (3):** 396 – 399.
31. Sejvar J.J. **Neurologic adverse events associated with smallpox vaccination in the United States 2002-2004.** *JAMA.* 2005, **294:** 2744 – 2750.
32. Hamidon B.B. Acute **disseminated encephalomyelitis (ADEM) presenting with seizures secondary to anti-tetanus toxin vaccination.** *Med. J. Malaysia.* 2003, **58 (5):** 780 – 782.
33. Jorge D. Machicado, Bhavana Bhagya-Rao, Giovanni Davogustto, Brandy J. McKelvy. Acute Disseminated Encephalomyelitis following Seasonal Influenza Vaccination in an Elderly Patient. ***Clinical and vaccine immunology,*** 2013, **20(9):** 1485-1486.
34. Pellegrino P, Carnovale C, Perrone V, Pozzi M, Antoniazzi S. et al. **Correction: Acute Disseminated Encephalomyelitis Onset: Evaluation Based on Vaccine Adverse Events Reporting Systems.** *PLoS ONE.* 2013, **8(12):** 10.1371.
35. Ann Yeh E. **Detection of coronavirus in the central nervous system of a child with acute disseminated encephalomyelitis.** *Pediatrics.* 2004, **113:** 73 – 76.
36. Tenembaum S. **Acute disseminated encephalomyelitis: a long-term follow-up study of 84pediatric patients.** *Neurology.* 2002, **22 (59 (8)):** 1224 – 1231.
37. Tenembaum S. **Disseminated encephalomyelitis in children.** *Clinical neurology and neurosurgery.* 2008, **110:** 928 – 938.
38. Alper G. Acute disseminated encephalomyelitis. *J Child Neurol,* 2012, **27(11):**1408-1425.
39. Krupp L.B. **International Pediatric Multiple Sclerosis Study Group 2007 Consensus definitions proposed for pediatric multiple sclerosis and related disorders.** *Neurology. –* 2007, **68 (16 suppl 2):** 7 – 12.
40. Sonneville R, T. Klein de Broucker J. **Post-infectious encephalitis in adults: Diagnosis and management.** *Infection. –* 2009, **58:** 321 – 328.
41. Ogava Y. **A case of acute disseminated encephalomyelitis presenting with vertigo.** *Auris Nasus Larynx.* 2008, **35:** 127 – 130.

42. Suppiej A, Vittorini R, Fontanin M. **Acute disseminated encephalomyelitis in children: focus on relapsing patients.** *Pediatr Neurol.* – 2008, **39 (1):** 12 – 17.
43. Lobanova I., Myalovitska O. **The Efficacy of Intravenous Immunoglobulin in the Treatment of Patients with Acute Disseminated Encephalomyelitis.** *Journal of Advances in Medical and Pharmaceutical Sciences.* 2015, **2(4):** 154-163.
44. Brass SD. **Multiple sclerosis and acute disseminated encephalomyelitis in childhood.** *Pediatr. Neurol.* 2003, **29(3):** 227 – 231.
45. McGovern RA, DiMario FJ. **Acute disseminated encephalomyelitis: a retrospective pediatric serie.** *Ann. Neurol.* 2003, **54 (7):** 127 – 129.
46. Neuteboom RF, Catsman-Berrevoets CE, Hintzen RQ. **Multiple sclerosis in children.** *Ned Tijdschr Geneeskd.* 2007, **151(26):** 1464 – 1468.
47. Pohl D, Hennemuth I, Kries R. **Paediatric multiple sclerosis and acute disseminated encephalomyelitis in Germany:results of a nationwide survey.** *Eur. J. Pediatr.* 2007, **166:** 405 – 412.
48. Toshiyuki O, Shunsaku H. **Reccurence of acute disseminated encephalomyelitis after a 12-year symptom-free interval.** *Interval Medicine.* 2004, **43(8):** 746 – 749.
49. Tur C, Téllez N, Rovira A. **Acute disseminated encephalomyelitis: study of factors involved in a possible development towards multiple sclerosis.** *Neurologia.* 2008, **23(9):** 546 – 554.
50. Polman CH, Reingold SC, Banwell B., Clanet M. et al. **Diagnostic criteria for multiple sclerosis: 2010 revisions to the ''McDonald Criteria''.** *Ann Neurol.* 2011, **69 (2):** 292–302.
51. Hung KL. **The spectrum of postinfectious encephalomyelitis.** *Brain Dev.* 2001, **23:** 42 – 45.
52. Anlar B. **Acute disseminated encephalomyelitis in children: outcome and prognosis.** *Neuropediatrics.* 2003, **34(4):** 194 – 199.
53. Huynh W, Cordato DJ, Kehdi E. **Post-vaccination encephalomyelitis: literature review and illustrative case.** *J. Clinical Neuroscience.* 2008: 1315 – 1322.
54. Mikaeloff Y, Caridade G, Husson B, et al. **Acute disseminated encephalomyelitis cohort study: prognostic factors for relapse.** *Eur. J. Paediatr. Neurol.* 2007, **11(2):** 90 – 95.
55. Dale RC, Sousa C, Chong WK. **Acute disseminated encephalomyelitis, multiphasic disseminated encephalomyelitis and multiple sclerosis in children.** *Brain.* 2000, **123:** 2407 – 2224.
56. Leake JA. **Acute disseminated encephalomyelitis in childhood: epidemiologic, clinical and laboratory features.** *Pediatr. Infect. Dis. J.* 2004, **23:** 756 – 764.

57.Cohen O. **Recurrence of acute disseminated encephalomyelitis at the previously affected brain site.** *Arch. Neurol.* 2001, **58:** 797 – 801.

58.Dale RC, Branson JA. **Acute disseminated encephalomyelitis or multiple sclerosis: can the initial presentation help in establishing a correct diagnosis.** *Arch. Dis. Child.* 2005, **90:** 636 – 639.

59.Divya SK, Mrlvin JJ, Sanjeev VK. **Acute disseminated encephalomyelitis in children: discordand neurologic and neuroimaging abnormalities and response to plasmapheresis.** *Pediatrics.* 2005, **166(2):** 431 – 436.

60.Kanter DS, Horensky D, Sperling RA. **Plasmapheresis in fulminant acute disseminated encephalomyelitis.** *Neurology.* 1995, **45:** 824 – 827.

61.Aboagye-Kumi M. et M. **ADEM in a renal thansplantationrecipient; a case report.** *Transplantation proceedings.* 2008, **40:** 1751-1753.

62.Khurana DS, Melvin JJ, Kothare SV. **Acute disseminated encephalomyelitis in children: discordant neurologic and neuroimaging abnormalities and response to plasmapheresis.** *Pediatrics.* 2005, **116(2):** 431 – 436.

63.Pohl D, Tenembaum S. Treatment of acute disseminated encephalomyelitis. *Curr Treat Options Neurol.* 2012, **14(3):** 264-75.

64.Ravaglia S. **Severe steroid-resisnant post-infectious encephalomyelitis: general features and effects of IVIg.** *J. Neurol.* 2007, **254 (11):** 1518 – 1523.

65.Shahar E. **Outcome of severe encephalomyelitis in children: effect of high-dose methylprednisolone and immunoglobulin.** *J. Child Neurol.* 2002, **17:** 810 – 814.

66.Sonneville R. **Acute disseminated encephalomyelitisin the intensive careunit: clinical features and outcome of 20 adults.** *Intensive Care Med.* 2008, **24 (3):** 528 – 532.

67.Tenembaum S. **Acute disseminated encephalomyelitis.** *Neurology.* 2007, **68:** 23 – 26.

68.Van Dam NC, Eron Syed S, Ostrander M. **Severe postvaccinal encephalitis with ADEM: recovery with early intravenous Ig, high-dose steroids and Vaccina Ig.** *Clinical infectious disease.* 2009. **48:** 47 – 49.

69.Fu DC, Montgomery JR. **High-dose, rapid-infusion IVIG in postvaccination acute disseminated encephalomyelitis.** *Neurology.* 2008, **71:** 294 – 295.

70.Joshua Rothenberg, Angie Lastra, Gemayaret Alvarez, Robert Irwin. **Acute Disseminated Encephalomyelitis Responsive to Cyclophosphamide Therapy: A Case Report.** *Journal of medical Cases,* 2015, **6 (7):** 290-294.

71.Kazushi Ichikawa, Hirotaka Motoi, Yoshitaka Oyama, Yoshihiro Watanabe, Saoko Takeshita. **Fulminant form of acute disseminated** encephalomyelitis in a child treated with mild hypothermia. *Pediatrics International,* 2013: e149–e151.

72. Kotlus BS, Slavin ML, Guthrie D. **Ophthalmologic manifestations in pediatric patients with acute disseminated encephalomyelitis.** *J AAPOS.* 2005, **9 (2):** 179 – 183.

73. Meca-Lallana JE. **Plasmaferesis: its use in multiple sclerosis and other demyelinating processes of the central nervous system. An oaservational study.** *Rev. Neurol.* 2003, **37:** 917 – 926.

74. Ohya T, Nagamitsu S, Yamashita Y. **Serial magnetic resonance imaging and single photon emission computed tomography study of acute disseminated encephalomyelitis patient after Japanese encephalitis vaccination.** *Kurume Med. J.* 2007, **54(3-4):** 95 – 99.

75. Berrak S., Seda Sirin Kose, Serdar Saritas, Engin Kose, Ali Kanik, Mehmet Helvaci. **Severe Acute Disseminated Encephalomyelitis With Clinical Findings of Transverse Myelitis After Herpes Simplex Virus Infection.** *J Child Neurol,* 2014, **29:** 1519-1523.

76. **Konstantin Huhn, De-Hyung Lee, Ralf A Linker, Stephan Kloska, Hagen B Huttner,** Corresponding author: Konstantin Huhn. **Pneumococcal-meningitis associated acute disseminated encephalomyelitis (ADEM) – case report of effective early immunotherapy.** *SpringerPlus,* 2014, **3:** 415.

77. Lu Z, Zhang B, Qiu W, Kang Z, Shen L, Long Y, et al. **Comparative Brain Stem Lesions on MRI of Acute Disseminated Encephalomyelitis, Neuromyelitis Optica, and Multiple Sclerosis.** *PLoS ONE.* 2011, **6(8):** e22766

78. Nishicava M, Ichiama T. **Intravenous immunoglobulin therapy in acute disseminated encephalomyelitis.** *Pediatr. Neurol.* 1999, **21(2):** 583 – 586.

79. Pittock SJ. **Rapid clinical and CSF response to intravenous gamma globulin in acute disseminated encephalomyelitis.** *Eur. J. neurology.* 2001, **8:** 723 – 725.

80. Shiraiwa N, Yoshizawa T, Ohkoshi N. **A case of acute disseminated encephalomyelitis (ADEM) associated with peripheralneuropathy.** *Rinsho Shinkeigaku.* 2007, **47 (4):** 169 – 172.

81. Straussberg R. **Improvement of atypical acute disseminated encephalomyelitis with steroids and intravenous immunoglobulins.** *Pediatric Neurology.* 2001, **24:** 139 – 143.

82. Sunnerhagen KS, Johansson K, Ekholm S. **Rehabilitation problems after acute disseminated encephalomyelitis.** *J. Rehabilitation Medicine.* 2003, **35:** 20 – 25.

83. Unay B. **Intravenous immunoglobulin therapy in acute disseminated encephalomyelitis associated with hepatitis A infection.** *Pediatr. Int.* 2004, **46 (2):** 171 – 173.

84. Varilek BZ, Eron Syed S, Ostrander M. **Acute disseminated encephalomyelitis following pleural empyema owing to Boerhaave's syndrome.** *J. Child Neurol.* 2004, **19 (3):** 224 – 227.

85. Laderman M, Gabelin P, Lafrenz M. **Acute disseminated encephalomyeltis malaria caused by Varicella Zoster Virus reactivation.** *Amer. J. Trop. Med. Hyg.* 2005, **72 (4):** 478 – 480.

86. Lin CH, Jeng JS, Yip PK. **Plasmapheresis in acute disseminated encephalomyelitis.** *J. Clin. Apher.* 2004, **19 (3):** 154 – 159.

87. Ramachandran NR, Parameswaran MG. **Acute disseminated encephalomyelitis treated with plasmapheresis.** *Singapore Med J.* 2005, **46 (10):** 561 – 563.

88. Ramachandran NR. **Plasmapheresis in childhood acute disseminated encephalomyelitis.** *Indian Pediatr.* 2005, **42(5):** 479 – 482.

89. Refai D. **Decompressive hemicraniectomy for acute disseminated encephalomyelitis.** *Neurosurgery.* 2005, **56(4):** 870 – 872.

90. Kurtzke JF. **Rating neurological impairment in multiple sclerosis: an expanded disability staty scale (EDSS).** *Neurology.* 1983, **3:**1444 – 1452.

91. Hahn CD. Miles BS, MacGregor DL. **Neurocognitive outcome after acute disseminated encephalomyelitis.** *Pediatr. Neurol.* 2003, 29 (2):117 – 123.

92. Delis DC, Kramer JH, Kaplan E, Ober BA. **The California Verbal Learning Test.** *San Antonio, TX: Psychological Corporation.* 1987.

93. Benedet MJ. Alejandre MA. **Test de aprendizaje verbal Espana-Complutense (TAVEC).** *TEA.* Madrid.

94. Folstein MF, Folstein SE, McHugh PR. **"Mini-mental state". A practical method for grading the cognitive state of patients for the clinician".** *Journal of Psychiatric Research.* 1975, **12 (3):** 189–98.

95. Bergner M, Bobbit R, Carter W, Gilson B. The Sickness Impact Profile: Development and Final Revision of a Health Condition Measure. Med Care. 1981, 8:787-805.

96. Simon J. Williams. **Measuring health condition? A review of the Sickness Impact and functional limitations profiles.** Health CARE ANALYSIS. 1996, **4(4):**273-283.

97. Kaplan EL, Meier P. No**nparametric estimation from incomplete observations.** *J. Amer. Statist. Assn.* 1958, 53:457–481.

98. Berwick V, Cheek L, Ball J. **Statistics review 12: Survival analysis.** *Crit Care.* 2004,**8:**389–94.

99. Azulay JP, Verschueren A, Attarian S. **Guillain-Barre syndrome and its frontiers.** *Rev. Neurol.* 2002, **158 (123):** 21 – 26.

100. Barohn RJ, Saperstein DS. **Guillain-Barre syndrome and chronic inflammatory demyelinating polyneuropathy.** *Semin. Neurol.* 1998, **18 (1):** 49 – 61.

101. De Grandis E, De Negri E, Montaldi L. **Intravenous immunoglobulins as therapeutic option in the treatment of multiple sclerosis.** *J. Neurol.* 2006, **253:** 50 – 58.

102. Gorson KC, Allam G, Ropper AH. **Chronic inflammatory demyelinating polyneuropathy: clinical features and response to treatment in 67 consecutive patients with and without a monoclonal gammopathy.** *Neurology.* 1997, **48 (2):** 321 – 328.

103. Smith-Jensen T, Burgoon, M, Anthony G, et al. **Comparison of IgG heavy chain sequences in MS and SSPE brain reveal an antigen-driven response.** *Neurology.* 2000, **54:** 1227 – 1232.

104. Takigawa T, Yasuda H, Terada M. **The sera from GM1 ganglioside antibody positive patients with Guillain-Barre syndrome or chronic inflammatory demyelinating polyneuropathy blocks Na+ currents in rat single myelinated nerve fibers.** *Intern. Med.* 2000, **39 (2):** 123 – 127.

105. Villa AM, Molina H, Sanz OP. **Chronic inflammatory demyelinating polyneuropathy. Findings in 30 patients.** *Medicina.* 1999, **59 (6):** 721 – 726.

106. Vital C, Vital A, Gbikpi-Benissan G. **Postvaccinal inflammatory neuropathy: peripheral nerve biopsy in 3 cases.** *J. Peripher. Nerv. Syst.* 2002, **7 (3):** 163 – 167.

107. Wittstock M, Zettl UK. **Adverse effects of treatment with intravenous immunoglobulins for neurological diseases.** *J Neurol.* 2006, **(5):** 75-79.

108. Basta M, Kirshbom P, Frank MM, Fries LS. **Mechanism of therapeutic effect of high-dose intravenous immunoglobulin. Attenuation of acute, complement-dependent immune damage in a guinea pig model.** *J Clin Invest* 1989, **(84):** 1974-1981.

109. Frank MM, Basta M, Fries LF. **The effects of intravenous immune globulin on complement dependent immune damage of cells and tissues.** *Clin Immunol Immunopathol.* 1992, **(62):** S82-S86.

110. Marchioni E, Marinou-Aktipi K, Uggetti C. **Efficacy of intravenous immunoglobulin treatment in adult patients with steroid-resistant monophasic or recurrent acute disseminated encephalomyelitis.** *J. Neurol.* 2002, **249 (1):** 100 – 104.

111. Giovanni SR, Ceroni PM. **Severe steroid-resistant post-infectious encephalomyelitis. General features and effects of IVIg.** *Neurol.* 2007, **254:** 1518 – 1523.

112.   Kleiman M, Brunquell P. **Acute disseminated encephalomyelitis: response to intravenous immunoglobulin.** *J Child Neurol.* 1995, **(10)**: 481-483.
113.   Shahar E. **Outcome of severe encephalomyelitis in children: effect of high-dose methylprednisolone and immunoglobulins.** *J. Child Neurol.* 2002, **(17)**: 810 – 814.
114.   Fazekas F., Lublin F.D., Li D., Freedman M.S. et al. **Intravenous immunoglobulin in relapsing-remitting multiple sclerosis. A dose-finding trial.** *Neurology*, 2008, **(71) 4:** 265-271.

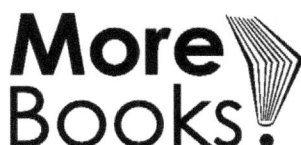
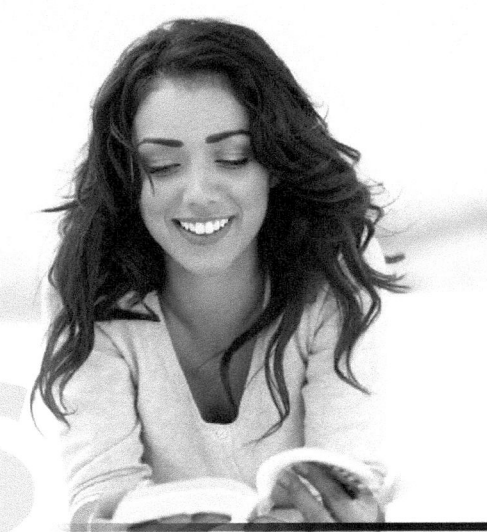
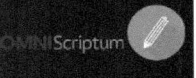

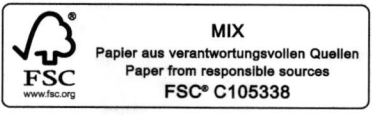
Printed by Books on Demand GmbH, Norderstedt / Germany